Overcoming Migraines and Other Headaches

'When the head aches, all the body is out of tune.'
From *Don Quixote*
by Miguel de Cervantes Saavedra

Headaches and migraines are a common and a distressingly painful disorder suffered silently by millions of healthy individuals. It afflicts all age groups, from the elderly to adolescents and infants with equal intensity and frequency, causing tremendous loss of personal and professional opportunities.

Headache is not a disease. It is a symptom. There are tension headaches and migraines (the two most common categories), cluster headaches, neuralgic headaches, and headaches associated with eye strain, hormonal changes, menopause, birth control pills, allergies, sinus, and even sex. Some headaches go away with little or no treatment. Others don't. This book will help you understand different types of headaches, identify your particular type, and what maybe causing it.

The book covers recent advances in medication and sophisticated control techniques. It also examines the role and importance of complimentary and non-medical therapies — homeopathy, acupuncture, diathermy, massage, hypnosis, and breathing techniques. Whatever the treatment, doctors agree that success depends largely on personal participation. This book will help in better understanding of the problems that accompany headaches and includes recommendations for daily living. It explains how certain changes in lifestyle — better nutrition, a little more exercise, a relaxed attitude — coupled with appropriate treatment, can control, reduce, and even eliminate the pain.

About the Authors

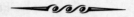

Joseph Kandel, M.D., is the founder and medical director of the Neurology Center of Naples in Naples, Florida, and cofounder of the Gulfcoast Spine Institute. An avid student since his youth, he attended Ohio State University as a Batelle Scholar, obtaining a double major B.S. in zoology and a B.S. in psychology, both with honors. Kandel graduated from Wright State University School of Medicine in Dayton, Ohio, in 1985, where he was president of his freshman medical school class. He completed his residency at the University of California Irvine Medical Center.

Kandel is a popular public speaker and has been published in such prestigious medical journals as *Neurology, Vital Signs,* and *American Zoologist.*

David Sudderth, M.D., is the senior partner at the Neurology Center of Naples and is cofounder of the Gulfcoast Spine Institute in Naples, Florida.

He graduated from medical school at the University of Copenhagen in 1984 and completed his residency at the Medical College of Wisconsin and Emory University. Dr. Sudderth accomplished a one-year fellowship in nerve and muscle disorders at Emory University in 1988.

An in-demand lecturer, Sudderth speaks frequently on medical topics. He also produced the popular video *Spinal Tips* and has published in *Neurology* and *Ugeskrift For Laeger.*

OVERCOMING
Migraines AND
OTHER
Headaches

Dr Joseph Kandel MD
Dr David Sudderth MD

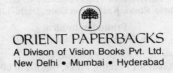

ORIENT PAPERBACKS
A Divison of Vision Books Pvt. Ltd.
New Delhi • Mumbai • Hyderabad

*To my wife, Merrylee, and our children, Max,
Hannah Rose, and Geena. Your love, patience,
and support made this work possible. And to my
parents, for their unending love.*

JOSEPH KANDEL

*To my friends, family, patients, and teachers,
without whose interest and encouragement this
work would not have been possible.*

DAVID B. SUDDERTH

ISBN 81-222-0228-4

Ist Published in Orient Paperbacks 1998

Overcoming Migraines and Other Headaches

© 1996 Joseph Kandel & David B. Sudderth

Cover design by Vision Studio

Published in arrangement with
Prima Communications, Inc., USA

Published by
Orient Paperbacks
(A division of Vision Books Pvt. Ltd.)
Madarsa Road, Kashmere Gate, Delhi-110 006

Printed in India at
Kay Kay Printers, Delhi-110 007

Cover Printed at
Ravindra Printing Press, Delhi-110 006

Contents

———∽∽∽———

Acknowledgements: Special thanks go to Chris Adamec for her extensive assistance. Also thanks to Betty Lavery for her dedicated persistence in transcription. We especially acknowledge Sue Felber for her insightful assistance in obtaining relevant resources for our research, and our devoted office staff for their patience during the writing and production of this book.

Introduction

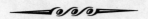

Migraine is a common, cruel, and pervasive disorder suffered by 23 million Americans, not only afflicting them with great pain but also robbing them of control over their personal, family, and work lives. The National Center for Health Statistics reports that migraine headaches result in a loss of 30 million work days costing the economy $4.5 billion per year. Further, no one could begin to accurately quantify the collective anguish and pain migraineurs suffer, as well as their loss of personal and professional opportunities. Yet today there is much hope for migraineurs thanks to new treatment and medication.

People have suffered from migraines since recorded time. The ancient Babylonians, Greeks, and Romans experienced migraines, and cavemen probably did, too. Famous individuals, including Thomas Jefferson, Alexander Pope, Dorothy Wordsworth, Ulysses S. Grant, and many others were migraine sufferers. According to Grant's own memoirs, one of his migraines evaporated upon the news of Lee's surrender.

The pain of these famous migraine sufferers of the past was no more intense than the suffering of today's enterprising computer programmer, civil servant, or any other individual with an agonizing migraine. But there is one difference: today physicians can alleviate much of that pain. It's rare for a neurologist to be completely unable to assist the patient with debilitating migraine headaches. As physicians, we are very optimistic about the prognosis for migraineurs, and you should be, too!

1

What Is a Migraine?

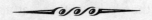

A migraine is a serious, debilitating, and often painful illness originating in the brain. The migraine may last for a few minutes or a few days—or for any period of time in between.

Subtypes of Migraine

Migraine headaches are divided into two major subtypes: the classic migraine and the common migraine. The key difference between the two is that the classic migraine follows an "aura," while a common migraine appears with no aura.

So what's an aura? The aura is a brief episode of symptoms that are related to a focal area of dysfunction in the brain and may include visual disturbances, dizziness, and other symptoms. The aura will be discussed in greater detail later in this chapter.

Sometimes people with classic migraine also suffer from common migraine. Getting one kind doesn't exempt you from getting the other form. Sorry!

In order to diagnose and treat migraines, we adhere to the headache classification committee guidelines of the International Headache Society.

Frequency of Occurrence

People who experience common migraine headaches usually suffer from one to four headaches per month. Yet about ten percent have ten or more migraines monthly, and some people have no more than two to three attacks of migraine in their entire lives.

Common migraine is seen more often by doctors, occurs more frequently, and lasts longer than does the classic migraine. Nausea and vomiting are also worse in the common migraine. All this doesn't necessarily mean that classic migraine is "better"—it's not the one you'd choose if you could pick one over the other. Classic migraine has its own scary elements, notably the aura aspect, which we'll discuss in a few pages.

Migraine Differs from Person to Person

One fact that may surprise you is that the onset and the course of the illness varies greatly among "migraineurs" (people who suffer from migraines), and some people—not very many!—don't even get a headache. This chapter discusses what actually happens to the body during an acute attack. Let's start off with an interesting but unusual case.

Anne B., 35, came to the office with very peculiar symptoms, primarily involving recurring "black eyes." She was mystified. The black eyes were spontaneous—they "just happened" and didn't seem to be associated with any other symptoms.

Intermittent headaches had been a serious problem for Anne for several years, but in the past twelve months, her headaches had changed and, unfortunately, had become considerably worse. These new headaches would begin as an aching type of headache and within thirty minutes would surge into excruciating pain, intense nausea, and vomiting.

Often the "raccoon eyes" were present the day after one of these severe headaches, although Anne said that the eye discoloration could occur before the headaches or even with no headache.

The black eye symptoms Anne experienced are only one of the many physical changes that may occur in a patient with migraine. We treated Anne with a moderate dose of Inderal along with intermittent Sumatriptan, and she has greatly improved with regard to her headache frequency and duration.

Profound alterations may also occur in the circulatory system, gastrointestinal function, and mental and emotional states of the patient. In fact, some of the phenomena witnessed in a migrainous attack belong to the most fascinating and exciting realm of human existence.

If you suffer from migraine, you probably know that this illness is enthralling to some medical observers and irksome and perplexing to others. You also know that the various features of the migraine attack can often lead to intense and excruciating misery in the patient. Some patients are driven into a desperate panic or a bewildered lethargic state.

The bottom line: It's no fun at all.

Prodrome

Sometimes migraineurs get a kind of advance warning of an impending migraine, a sort of "yellow light" alert, which is called the "prodrome."

A prodrome is different from an aura because the prodromal symptoms may be very vague and begin slowly, with great variation in how long they last. Vague warnings of an impending headache often precede either the headache or the aura, and if sufferers can take immediate action, they may be able to stop the migraine cold—or at least beat it back to a bearable level.

Prodromes occur more frequently than the aura itself does. Comments such as "I don't feel myself today" and "I feel like a train hit me"—along with many other remarks ranging between both extremes—are common from migraineurs prior to the onslaught of their headaches. It should also be emphasized here that occasionally a prodrome will not develop into a full-blown migrainous attack.

Changes in mood are common prodromal symptoms; for example, patients may feel very depressed and lethargic. But sometimes, they actually feel a sense of increased well-being and a high energy level. But watch out! Bad times lie ahead as the migraine comes on like a speeding bullet.

Felix S., 32, our patient for several years, was diagnosed as having common migrainous attacks, which were fairly well controlled with Inderal. The additional use of injectable Sumatriptan has greatly helped reduce the severity of his attacks.

Felix says that he always knew when a headache was coming the second he opened his eyes in the morning. He could barely lift himself out of bed, and once he was finally out, he was intensely irritable. His family knew to stay out of his way.

The Aura

Migraine sufferers may also experience a range of symptoms classified under an experience known as the "aura."

The aura is a brief episode of symptoms that are related to a focal area of dysfunction in the brain. In general, an aura lasts less than twenty minutes and usually appears before the head pain begins. However, the aura can recur at various points of the headache, such as during the most intensely painful point.

Auras may be simple (migraineurs see flashing lights, wavy lines, etc.) or have the character of a complex hallucinatory experience—truly frightening. However, once the nature of the aura has been carefully explained to and understood by the migraineur, its more horrifying aspects can be dispelled.

Visual Aura

Visual auras are the most common among those who experience any form of aura. The more simple visual disturbance is the "photopsia," which consists of circles, triangles, squares, or other geometric patterns, usually white or multicolored. Typically, the person sees these figures in any part of the visual field, and they may move about. Although not really there, the patterns are clearly "seen" by the migraineur. This may be due to irritation to the vision center of the brain and probably has nothing to do with either eye.

Sometimes more complex and symmetrical patterns are occasionally seen. These visual disturbances may occur even if the person is blind or both eyes have been physically removed. Here is one description given by a migraine sufferer, quoted by Sacks in the medical book, *Migraine— Evolution of a Common Disorder* (University of California Press, 1970).

> a bright stellate object, a small angled sphere suddenly appears in one side of the combined field . . . it rapidly enlarges . . . and, as the increase in size goes on, the outline here becomes broken, the gap becoming larger as the hole increases, and the original circular outline

becomes oval . . . when this angled oval has extended through the greater part of the half-field the upper portion expands; it seems to overcome at least some resistance in the immediate neighborhood of the fixing point . . . so that a bulge occurs in the part above, and the angular elements of the outline here enlarge. . . . This final expansion near the centre progresses with great rapidity, and ends a whirling centre of light from which sprays of light seem flying off. Then all is over, and the headache comes on.

That sounds bad enough, but some patients have also reported truly complex and bizarre visual disturbances—so unsettling they were reluctant to report them to their doctors unless specifically asked about them. Why? Probably because they feared their doctors would consider them mentally ill. But neurologists are very familiar with this problem and need to be told what's going on so they can help you.

Another example of visual aura is when an object is seen as extremely distorted, much like images and proportions are distorted in a funhouse mirror. An Alice in Wonderland experience can occur where suddenly a person may appear to have an elongated neck or someone's head may appear dramatically larger while the legs looks disproportionately small.

Changes in distance perceptions may occur, too—how close or how far away objects appear to be may be completely out of alignment with reality. Think of the warning on the sideview mirror on some cars: "Objects in mirror are closer than they appear." Then magnify that ten times or more.

Disorders of sensation and movement are the next most common features of a classic aura. Often the sensation may involve a feeling of numbness on one side of the face, usually the mouth, and also in the hand and arm on the same side of the body. These symptoms tend to develop within thirty minutes and can terrify the patient, who is convinced that he or she is in the middle of a stroke or maybe even dying.

Weakness or clumsiness in the arms and legs often occur as part of the aura. Sometimes pain in a limb is the primary feature of an aura.

Other Types of Aura

Dizziness or abnormal sensations of motion are well-documented features of an aura. Other hallucinatory experiences can consist of auditory misperceptions, such as a ringing or crackling noise in the ears.

Sometimes patients will lose the ability to speak (aphasia), although comprehension of spoken language usually is not lost. Or they may experience an olfactory hallucination, where they smell something that is not there. Fortunately, both aphasia and olfactory hallucinations are rarely reported. Often migraineurs have a sensation of "deja vu," that they are re-experiencing feelings or sensations exactly as they have in the past.

In one reported case, a 38-year-old man who suffered from severe migraines also usually experienced amnesia during the attacks. However, at one point he reported that he did remember seeing gray Indians, 20 centimeters high, crowding around him in his room. This most likely represented an irritation in the part of the brain that handles memory. Such an irritation affects certain fibers that pass through this area carrying or triggering vision sensations.

The Headache

The headache can be absent altogether, or it can be so agonizingly painful that the patient seriously contemplates suicide. Often the headache is on one side (called hemicranial—

half of the head), but it can occur on both sides of the head. Sometimes the sides even switch! The left side could suddenly become pain-free and then the right side is in agony (or vice versa). Headaches that occur on only one side seem to be more painful.

The initial pain of a migraine is often described as vise-like or of a pressing, gripping nature that may later progress to a throbbing, banging, or pounding headache.

The migrainous head pain can be localized to anywhere on the face or scalp and can even affect the structures of the upper portion of the neck. Usually, the frontal (forehead) regions are affected, as well as the eye area.

Pain may affect the person's entire skull, and the scalp itself is often very tender during a migrainous attack. Sometimes the migraine is confined to the lower area of the face below the eyes and is called a lower-half migraine.

Most migraines last from one to three hours, although children sometimes experience headaches of less than ten minutes.

The migraine is so devastating to the body that few sufferers can think of anything but the pain and suffering. In addition, activities which increase the pressure inside the brain—such as sneezing, coughing, or vomiting—can be agonizingly painful to the patient. Often migraineurs press on the pulsating arteries in front of their ears, trying to control the pain. This usually doesn't work.

Other Symptoms

If cigarette smoke or perfume bothers you when you have a migraine, you are not alone. Often virtually any odor is intolerable to migraineurs, and strong odors can increase the physical pain of the headache.

Sometimes loud noises disturb the person with a migraine; this is often referred to as phonophobia. No drumrolls, please, and make your teenager use his headphones.

Likewise, bright lights or even routine daylight can increase your pain. This is called photophobia.

Nausea and Vomiting

About half of all patients suffer from nausea and vomiting. Sometimes the arrival of nausea signals that the head pain will abate; however, it could also mean the pain is going to get worse! The significance of nausea and vomiting truly varies from person to person, and people who suffer from migraines learn what it means from their own experience. Generally, nausea signals that things are going to get better or they're going to get worse, rather than stay the same.

Sometimes the vomiting is so severe or the person sweats so much that he or she loses too much fluid and needs intravenous therapy to replace the loss of water and sodium. Conversely, sometimes fluid is retained in the body.

Gastrointestinal changes include diarrhea or constipation and abdominal cramps. In addition to these abdominal changes, one of the most significant aspects migraine sufferers experience is that, at the time of an acute attack, the stomach can actually become paralyzed. That's right, they can encounter what's called "gastroparesis," which complicates the migraine even more by preventing medicines taken by mouth from being effective. Since oral medications have to go through the stomach to work, it makes sense that other forms of intervention may be necessary. This is an all-too-often overlooked aspect of migraine management, particularly by physicians who are not comfortable providing care to migraineurs.

Intervention in the form of medications by nasal spray, rectal suppository, or injection may become the medication of choice to abort an acute migraine, particularly if the migraine has been present for more than thirty to sixty minutes. This is the approximate time frame it takes for the stomach to become sluggish or even stop absorbing chemicals, nutrients, and medications.

Circulatory Changes

In the beginning of this chapter, we described the patient with the "raccoon eyes," which apparently resulted from circulatory changes associated with her migraines.

More frequently, we see patients who are very pale, except for flushing that may be seen on one side of the face—the hurting side. Sometimes the dilation of blood vessels is so severe that it causes actual hemorrhage (severe bleeding) in the nose area, or superficially in the eyeballs.

Increased blood flow in the mucous membranes of the nose can also cause nasal congestion, drooping eyelids, and changes in eye pupil sizes. It can lead to sinus congestion and is often related to that stuffy sensation of the nose, which can be confused with sinusitis.

The patient may insist that he or she has a fever when there is no fever, while others complain they feel cold and clammy, especially in their hands and feet.

The heart rate may increase or decrease in this multifaceted illness.

Changes in Behavior

If the greatest and most heartfelt wish of the migraineur is relief from headache, the second greatest wish is for seclusion. Just leave them alone!

Unlike patients with kidney stones or cluster headaches, who characteristically rush about or leave home seeking relief, the migraineur will generally choose an immobile position. Usually migraine victims will lie down, although they may sit or stand very still.

Patients in the throes of an uncomfortable attack are generally very irritable, although some may be passive. People who are normally even-tempered, kind, and loving individuals can be transformed into stubborn, rude, and extremely insensitive creatures.

One patient told us that during an attack, he looked like a wax statue, felt like a martyr, and behaved like Satan himself.

Sometimes people with migraine become extremely drowsy and all they want to do is sleep. It's not a good idea to try to wake them up! Let sleeping migraineurs lie.

Mental ability can even be affected by a migraine. Patients with migraines generally perform more poorly than they normally would on tests requiring higher-ordered processes such as mathematical thought, concentration, or creative activity. In addition, memory lapses may occur, and the unhappy and perplexed migraineur may later be confronted with things he or she said or did during an attack—but doesn't remember at all.

Sometimes behavioral changes are extreme, and in very rare cases can even be psychotic. For example, the patient may feel a sense of unreality or may become violent and uncontrollable and need to be restrained, either chemically or physically. Patients who react in this way during migraine episodes usually don't remember what happened during the attack.

It's Over . . . For Now

As the migraine subsides and ends, most patients state that they still don't feel "right." Often, they complain of a lack of initiative, a kind of mental dullness or cloudiness and a generalized weakness. One patient said she feels "like a zombie" after an attack. After such a massive assault on the body that some migraine headaches cause, this reaction is certainly not surprising.

So far we have attempted to describe the symptoms of migraine from the simple to the complex. What type of process can lead to such a bizarre and variable collection of symptoms? In the next chapter, we will explore the leading theories offered to account for this truly perplexing disorder.

2

Theories of Migraine:
What Causes Them?

⟿⟾

What actually causes people to suffer from migraine headaches? Physicians aren't entirely sure, but they do have theories for the basic causes. Most doctors generally select from four primary theories.

You don't need to become a medical doctor to understand these theories, and it's a good idea to learn what physicians believe is the likely cause of your problem. Why? Because knowledge is power, and the more you understand your own body and your reactions to food and medications, the more you are empowered to combat the insidious problem of migraine headaches.

One type of migraine, basilar migraine, can actually appear as a coma. Therefore, it is important for your doctor to understand the variety of migraine disorders and how they are manifest. This knowledge will often provide clues to help determine what underlies the migraine.

We can classify theories of migraine causes as:

- Vascular
- Neural

- Neurovascular (a combination of neural and vascular)
- Neurochemical transmission/depletion theory

The Vascular Theory of Migraine

Clinicians who support the vascular theory believe that a migraine headache results directly from the expansion and contraction of blood vessels, both inside *and* outside the brain. When blood vessels dilate outside the brain, says this theory, this causes the blood vessels inside the brain to constrict.

Along with the narrowing of the blood vessels inside the brain comes a decreased blood flow and diminished oxygen flow to structures inside your brain. As a result of these changes, neurological symptoms such as migraines occur. Or so the theory goes.

Over the past decade, research has documented actual changes in blood flow during both the prodrome and onset of a migraine episode. Initially, with the spasm of blood vessels, there is also a change in the blood flow to the brain, and the migraine aura theoretically results from this spasm.

Then the blood dilations expand, and a release of numerous chemicals, known as vasoactive substances, occurs. This release is often associated with the "pounding" sensation from which migraine patients suffer.

The sequence continues, as the release of those vasoactive substances apparently triggers some central mechanism that lowers the pain threshold. That means it hurts you more than it would otherwise because your pain tolerance is decreased.

Additional evidence and anecdotal references do support the "pulsing temples," referring to the blood vessels over the forehead. These do actually appear to pulsate in a number of patients during a migraine episode.

In further support, in some cases, migraines can be treated by firm pressure over the temples, and some physicians have suggested constricting headband-like devices as curative.

More recently, using a device called a transcranial doppler (which monitors blood flow through the brain and arteries), researchers have found that the speed of blood flow in the middle cerebral artery decreases during a migraine attack. Somehow, your brain turns on the "yellow light" and the blood flow slows down, which is bad for migraineurs.

Further support for this theory comes from the fact that, in many cases, medications used to treat or prevent migraines specifically act by affecting the blood vessel wall stability. Such medications include beta blockers: Inderal, Tenormin, and Corgard. In addition, first-line medications for treating migraines have included calcium channel blockers such as Calan SR, Procardia, and Cardizem, which may act in a similar way.

Research done in 1995, using very specialized techniques of blood flow measurement, has revealed that during classic migraine, there is a region of a progressive decrease in blood flow. This is a key to the blood flow theory of migraine, and draws a relationship to migraines and "ischemic" strokes (related to lack of blood and oxygen).

Other researchers have concluded that there may be some association between the blood flow events of migraine and a future connection with the loss of blood and oxygen to the brain, resulting in stroke. The results were not clear-cut, but certainly do lend credence to the vascular theory of migraine disorder.

The Neural Theory

The neural hypothesis takes a slightly different approach to the causes of migraine headache disorders. Supporters of this theory believe that a migraine is actually a dysfunction of the nervous system and an unstable threshold in the brain.

When internal or external stressors increase, this threshold is exceeded, and a migraine headache is produced. It's sort of like one part of your body says "don't step over this line," but you do anyway, and suffer the consequences (all unconsciously, of course!).

This theory also seems to rely on a belief that there is a genetic predisposition for migraine headache disorders. It is true that migraine sufferers often have a strong family history of migraine. To further the theory of a genetic predisposition toward migraine, one sophisticated study found that a location on chromosome 19 was related to a unique type of migraine.

Another aspect of the neural theory is the belief that migraine is comprised of a unique constellation of symptoms, one of which is often misdiagnosed since it is too tough for the average primary care doc to call.

It's believed, as part of this theory, that migraine results from an irregular or abnormal nervous system outflow, a burst of electric energy, which can kindle or trigger a variety of areas in the brain. This subsequently produces a variety of symptoms, sort of like a microscopic lightning strike inside your brain.

As a result, many diverse symptoms may occur, such as severe headache associated with nausea and vomiting. Hallucinations may also occur, including imagined sights, sounds, tastes, or even smells. In addition, the patient may experience a variation of migraine that is also associated with abdominal queasiness often referred to as "abdominal migraine."

This theory also explains changes in mood or behavior, such as an essentially untriggered sense of elation, depression, anger, increased or decreased libido, or hunger—all of which can be symptoms of irritation in various parts of the brain.

In addition, imbalance and unsteadiness and even weakness and numbness can often be ascribed to atypical migraines.

Documented studies have also revealed that during the migraine phase, there are imbalances of glucose mechanism in different parts of the brain, suggesting that various parts of the brain are "selectively vulnerable" for certain people. This may explain why there is a tendency for one side of the head versus the other to become involved during migraine attacks.

In "complicated migraine," patients may present with weakness, numbness, language or speech dysfunction, and clumsiness and unsteadiness, depending on which parts of the brain are affected at a given time. These episodes can often mimic stroke symptoms and confuse physicians who are not neurologists. Yet, when the episode has subsided, within minutes to hours the neurological symptoms disappear as well.

As an example, psychiatrists have used the concept of "kindling" to explain causes of major depression. Frequently, the theory goes, there is irritation of a specific part of the brain (usually the temporal lobes) that can explain behavioral changes.

Similarly, once one part of the brain is kindled or the threshold is dropped, then other parts of the brain can likewise also become irritable, and thus trigger chemical changes of the brain.

The Neurovascular Theory

Supporters of this theory take a combination approach, believing that during attacks migraineurs have both abnormal or unstable blood vessels combined with a nervous system irritability.

It appears that much of the skull or facial pain that patients experience during migraine is carried along the distribution of the trigeminovascular pathways. (The trigeminal nerve is located near the cheekbone.) A possible defect in the chemical discharge along this pathway appears to be what causes the problem.

Think of this pathway as the highway where messages of pain are sent through the brain stem and into the sensory receptor (thalamus) part of the brain.

The result of stimulation can be that additional messages are sent to areas of the brain that interpret pain. So various parts of your brain are all saying "I feel pain!" And you do.

Combined with this is the problem that the intracranial blood vessels become unstable, with subsequent spasm and expansion of the blood vessels. The spasm, which is actually a protective mechanism to alter blood flow within your brain, can produce the changes associated with a lack of blood and oxygen. This is often referred to as the "migraine aura" and thus is how the supporters of this theory explain the aura.

Taking this theory a little further, the messages, which are carried up through the brain stem fibers to the thalamus and on to the cerebral cortex (the thinking part of the brain), are then associated with a spreading wave of chemical changes throughout your thinking center. This is often referred to as the "spreading depression" of migraine. Depending on the size of the region involved, various neurological signs and symptoms may occur.

This theory does seem to explain why a small number of patients have a multitude of symptoms without the clear-cut headache of migraine. In fact, which area of the brain is involved with this spreading depression apparently affects which symptoms a patient may experience.

For example, if the motor cortex were affected, then a patient might be weak or clumsy in an arm or leg or one side of the body only. On the other hand, if the frontal lobe regions became involved, a patient may feel confused, disoriented. and experience impaired judgment, feeling like he or she is "in a fog."

This unified hypothesis has been supported by various clinical studies, which have also revealed that a number of chemicals play a role in the brain stem function, including serotonin and acetylcholine—although serotonin is probably the major player.

In a Domino-like effect, activation of nerve cells in a region of the brain stem (the locus ceruleus), as well as in the dorsal raphe nuclei of the brain stem, apparently triggers a response in the nerve cells and the supporting structures and blood vessels of the region. All these responses taken together trigger an inflammatory response within the brain tissue itself, often through the trigeminal vascular pathways.

Throughout this whole process of body reactions and changes, there also appears to be a rebound effect, which seems to continue with the pain/inflammatory response. Compare it to a floodgate opening up. Not just one drop of water drips out, but instead all the water in the dam pours out.

Similarly, once the neurovascular system is inflamed, the neurochemicals or vasoactive substances that are released can continue a cycle of allowing the brain stem and thalamus to acknowledge pain and irritability, thereby keeping up the pain syndrome long after the external cause has been removed.

Since trigger causes are an important part of this theory, physicians who support it believe that patients should try to avoid those substances that apparently trigger migraine within their bodies. Some commonly known triggers are certain foods, such as cheese, citrus fruits, or chocolate, and some chemical food additives such as MSG.

In addition, stress, heat, infections, fumes, hormonal changes, and menstrual cycles can trigger migraines.

Note: Of course, hormonal changes and menstrual cycles are not so easily avoided. Some physicians have suggested women who suffer from migraine headaches during menstruation can mitigate the problem by taking an NSAID medication for five days before the cycle and also during the cycle. Others recommend that the patient take amitriptyline or propranolol during their menses. There is also some evidence that percutaneous estradiol gel just before and during menstruation can reduce the incidence of migraines.

Other triggers can be lack of sleep, too much sleep, or missing a meal. Drugs, including alcohol, can be powerful triggers for migraines. Weather changes can also trigger a migraine headache.

Neurochemical Transmission/ Depletion: The Serotonin Theory

A growing volume of research literature supports the role of impaired communication (neurotransmission) between brain cells (neurons). The brain is a telecommunications system *par excellence*, relying not only on electrical events but chemical occurrences as well to modulate the behavior of other cells. Serotonin is one of the many chemical neurotransmitters involved in intercellular communication (communication between brain cells). The serotonin-mediated chemical pathways are clearly implicated in the perception of pain.

Possibly the most supportive evidence is patient response to medications affecting serotonin. Many patients experience great relief from migraines by taking medications that directly affect serotonin levels, most notably Imitrex.

Researchers have recorded decreased blood levels of serotonin during migraine episodes, and urine concentrations of serotonin breakdown products seems to increase, so it is clear that there are serotonin changes in the body during a migraine headache. Some medications can also cause migraines. It appears as though medications that may reduce the circulating volume of serotonin may indeed trigger migraine episodes.

Additional support for this theory is that there are serotonin receptors in the stomach lining, which may explain why nausea and vomiting sometimes occur during an acute migraine attack.

Research in the 1970s and 1980s also revealed that implanting electrodes in the brain stem could produce migraine-like symptoms that lasted for days, weeks, months, or years. (Those poor research rats!) This coincides with the high concentration of serotonin receptors, which are presumed to control and modulate pain.

There are actually four different kinds of serotonin receptors. (Don't worry—we won't get too technical here!) Class one serotonin receptors appear to affect smooth muscle relaxation and smooth muscle contraction.

Class two serotonin receptors affect the discharge of nerve cells, the tightening of blood vessels, as well as some of the contraction to the airways in the lungs and the stomach wall.

Class three lead to activation of autonomic reflexes as well as to some nerve cell excitation in the brain and spinal cord.

Class four affect the stomach wall, heart stimulation, and relaxation of the food tube.

The serotonin theory explains why certain medications act on serotonin receptor one to block migraine episodes and relieve symptoms, while other medications work better on serotonin receptor two and so on.

Some people, especially holistic practitioners, are quick to point out that trace mineral changes in the body, vitamin deficiencies, and borderline nutrient deficiencies can all lead to severe migraine disorders. These practitioners approach headache disorders from that standpoint.

We feel that a combined theory of neurochemical changes (with an underlying genetic predisposition) lead to the cascade effect and the dumping of chemical changes in the brain, which lead to a vascular process—these best explain migraine now. This means that chemicals such as serotonin, norepinephrine, acetylcholine, GABA, and glutamate, among the many chemical messengers of the brain, reach some level of imbalance.

When the floodgates open, these chemicals irritate the blood vessels, and thus blood flow is altered. This change leads to the spreading change in oxygen and nutrients to various parts of the brain and explains the multitude of problems that migraine sufferers may experience. Depending upon which area of the brain is most vulnerable, we can see a variety of symptoms.

It is important to point out that when more than one theory exists regarding any medical problem, it means that no absolute answers are yet known. For example, in 1995, a new theory of migraine regarding a new tissue was proposed and reported in a popular magazine.

This tissue, heretofore unnoticed by physicians, was found at the base of the skull. The tissue was found by two dentists who were looking at causes of jaw pain and ended up cutting the skull of a cadaver at peculiar angles. Because of the change in dissection technique, this new tissue was discovered! The presumption is that this tissue, which is directly adjacent to the brain covering, can become very inflamed and can then trigger many responses, which in turn lead to headache pains similar to migraine disorder.

This is exciting, because it reveals that we are constantly gaining new information about how our bodies work and hopefully will eventually be able to put this information into one cohesive theory to explain the cause of migraine headache disorders.

Mechanism of Migraine Headache Disorder

The mechanism of migraine headache disorder formation is an additional important concept of how migraines are produced. The theory, backed up by scientific studies, is that the migraine can be caused by a deficiency of certain trace elements and minerals.

As we discuss elsewhere in this book, such things as deficiency in magnesium are often related to severe migraine pains. Thus treatment with either magnesium through the vein or magnesium replacement by mouth can lead to reduction or complete cessation of the migraine headache. While this does not give the absolute mechanism, one can infer that deficiencies affect the chemical change either in the brain or on the blood vessel wall and therefore act as a gatekeeper for toxins.

When the deficiencies of magnesium or other trace minerals and elements are not available to your body, the natural gatekeeper is not there and thus toxins and pollutants can trigger a migraine headache disorder. We are learning new information regarding magnesium and other minerals and elements every day, and this gives hope for the future of new and rational approaches to the management of migraine headache pain.

Recently, new information has come to light about headaches as one symptom of a larger disease. For example, patients who have had liver transplants may actually suffer from a new onset of migraines. While these patients had been susceptible to underlying medical processes, such as hypertension, infections, and other illnesses due to the medications they had taken, they also developed a migraine headache syndrome.

Research on this phenomenon may reveal to us that there is a systemic connection with the different organ systems, and that these organ systems are tied in together into a feedback system for the central nervous system (brain, spinal cord, etc.).

What this means is that when one organ system is unwell, it may trigger a negative response and produce illness in other organ systems. This then may be the mechanism which is at play in patients who have had liver transplants and suffer new onset migraine disorders.

Sometimes it's difficult for physicians to diagnose migraines. Or what they do diagnose as a migraine headache is in fact another form of head pain.

3

Chronic Daily Headache and Other Causes of Headache Pain: If It's Not Migraine, Then What Is It?

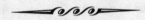

This chapter is one of the most important of this book. We will discuss the phenomenon of chronic daily headaches, which is a particularly distressing syndrome experienced by many migraine sufferers. We will also discuss some of the recent, disturbing reports about serious hazards of chronic use of over-the-counter medications.

Since there is some confusion between chronic daily headaches and migraine, a careful diagnosis is important. Remember, patients don't report in to the neurologist's office with the diagnosis "migraine" indelibly stamped on their foreheads. Instead, it takes the doctor some time, testing, and good professional judgment to make a determination.

The conditions discussed in this chapter are only the primary diagnostic entities that a qualified headache practitioner will consider in terms of a headache severe enough to warrant medical evaluation. Many are of a benign nature, but others can cause death.

Commonly recognized headache syndromes include muscle contraction headaches; temporomandibular joint dysfunction; neck disorders; trigeminal neuralgia; occipital neuralgia; eye disease; pseudotumor cerebri; cluster headaches; head trauma; temporal arteritis; tumors; abnormal blood vessels; stroke; and toxic states.

Chronic Daily Headaches

The chronic daily headache syndrome is a particularly distressing consequence of poorly treated migraine. While most neurologists are very familiar with this syndrome, many other physicians who treat migraine are grievously ignorant concerning the cause, nature, and treatment of this syndrome.

The syndrome consists of frequent headaches, usually for more than twenty days per month, in which the patient suffers from severe prostrating headaches, often accompanied by other common features of migraine. The pain can be entirely debilitating and lead to dehydration and utter despair in the patient.

The syndrome develops in an insidious manner. For example, migraineurs frequently have other types of headaches besides their migraines. They tend to use their anti-migrainous medications to deal with the other headaches that occur more often.

Initially, these headaches tend to respond to the medication. But then greater amounts of the drug are required over time to have the same effect. The medication in question can be ergotamine, acetaminophen, aspirin, or many of the other medications used for migraine, including those containing the barbiturate butalbital.

As the medication wears off, a very predictable headache appears: the chronic daily headache pattern. Interestingly, this type of headache pattern does not occur in non-migraineurs who actually take similar amounts and types of medication. For example, the syndrome is virtually unknown in patients suffering solely from cluster headaches or in arthritic patients who take large amounts of these medications.

It has also been shown from various studies that the antidepressant amitriptyline (Elavil), which is of great benefit as a preventive medication, is rendered ineffective in this context—more isn't better for the migraineur with daily headaches. Yet once the cycle of nearly daily headaches is broken, amitriptyline again becomes quite helpful in preventing not only migraines, but the other headaches from which migraineurs frequently suffer.

The severity and devastation of this daily type of headache cannot be overemphasized. Frequently, the patient is depressed and desperate by the time the condition is recognized, as well as totally unable to withstand detoxification on an outpatient basis. Often, it will be the patient himself who recognizes the situation and subsequently seeks relevant therapy.

For the patient who is suffering severe headaches and is not able to function professionally or socially, and in whom depression has become a factor, hospitalization is recommended. It should be noted that this syndrome can develop with even fairly small amounts of aspirin or acetaminophen of no more than 1000 to 1500 mg per day.

Treatment

While most patients initially resist the idea of hospitalization for something so "trivial" as headache, they frequently can be convinced of the necessity for this based on their degree of disability. Several studies have disagreed concerning the effectiveness of hospitalization, but many studies have validated this as a long-term solution for over half the patients who complete the therapy.

The goals of the therapy are fairly simple. The medications must be completely withdrawn as soon as possible and the various symptoms of the withdrawal state should be treated as effectively as possible.

Of course, not all medications *can* be safely withdrawn abruptly, including ergotamine, butalbital, and the various narcotics.

What happens during this withdrawal experience? The initial forty-eight hours are generally unpleasant for the patient. Many times, the patient experiences symptoms of an extremely bad migrainous attack. The nausea may be overwhelming, and the patient may experience vomiting to the point of dehydration and severe chemical imbalances. For this reason, intravenous feeding (IV) is frequently given during the first forty-eight hours.

The nausea is often controlled with anti-emetics such as prochlorperazine (Compazine) or metoclopramide (Reglan). Intravenous DHE 45 and methysergide have also proven quite helpful in this context.

After the first forty-eight hours, the patient will begin to recover, and a new course of treatment can be planned—one which does not rely solely on the medications that ultimately made the patient sicker.

Psychotherapy will often play a role in rehabilitating these patients, although it should be remembered that these patients did not begin using medications to achieve some sort of euphoric "high." Instead, they began taking the medications to relieve their headaches or their fear of these headaches. Depression, psychological trauma, and other psychological factors can of course influence the patient's analgesic abuse and should be dealt with appropriately.

Does Withdrawal Work?

Not all physicians agree that this regimen is effective, but studies do indicate a good response. Silverstein and Silverstein (1992) have reported that 87 percent of the patients completing detoxification remain free of analgesic abuse at a two-year follow-up after their release from hospital care.

Differential Diagnoses:
So What Else Could It Be?

Below we will describe the more common and recognized headache syndromes. We must emphasize that a complete list of all types of headaches would be beyond the scope of this book.

Tension Headaches

Tension headaches, also called muscle contraction headaches, are the most common type of headache. Few people have escaped experiencing this problem at some point in life. As the name suggests, the tension headache is frequently associated with some type of psychological distress. The headaches are thought to be related to increased tension in the scalp muscles.

Most portions of the skull are covered with a layer of muscle. Contraction in these muscles leads to reduced blood flow and presumably results in the tension headache. Generally, there is tenderness about the cranium during these headaches.

The tension headache is frequently described as a "tight band" about the head or almost a "viselike" sensation. The headache may be a throbbing pain and sufferers may even report nausea and vomiting—some neurologists have said that this indicates there is a continuum between muscle contraction headaches and migraine headaches.

Although the psychological aspect of these headaches is emphasized, they can occur without severe psychological stress or underlying psychological issue.

There is no threat to life, nor is there any prolonged disability associated with the tension headache. It usually responds to medication. We educate our patients about the distinction between this and migraine, and often suggest proper body movements to avoid increased neck muscle stress and spasm. (See "Activities for Daily Living" in the Appendix.)

In addition, it is often helpful to do directed neck exercises (see "Neck Knowledge and Neck Exercises" in the Appendix) to reduce pain and increase flexibility and range of motion. This can frequently prevent exacerbations and future flare-ups.

Temporomandibular Joint Dysfunction (TMJ)

Only in the most recent decade have mainstream physicians accepted the TMJ syndrome as a problem that causes headaches. This resistance toward acknowledging TMJ as a headache cause may be due to the absence of abnormalities on diagnostic tests such as magnetic resonance imaging (MRI). Grinding or clenching of the teeth (bruxism) at night and gum chewing are often found with individuals who have TMJ. Generally, the pain is in the temporal region as well as the jaw area itself. An advanced TMJ syndrome can lead to severe difficulties in speaking and in chewing.

This type of headache syndrome responds well to splints, medication, and physical therapy. Severe TMJ syndromes can require surgeries, which, unfortunately, rarely succeed.

Neck Pain

We have found that head pain frequently is accompanied by neck pain that is often of a degenerative joint type (arthritic or disc disease). Although headache resulting from a neck disorder can occur without neck pain, this rarely happens; you usually get both.

The site of the pain is typically in the back of the head near the neck area. Tenderness is common. The joints of the neck spine often become inflamed, and these can act as a powerful pain source called a facet syndrome.

Sinusitis

The sinuses are located behind the nose at the base of the forehead and below the eye sockets. Infection in any of these areas will cause localized pain. Usually, there will be marked tenderness over the sinuses in the forehead or below the eye sockets. Post nasal drip (mucous collection in the throat when lying on the back) commonly accompanies this problem.

More advanced cases of sinusitis are usually associated with fever and a general sensation of being ill. If not treated properly, this condition can escalate and lead to infections of the brain or its covering membranes (meningitis, which we also describe in this chapter).

Sinusitis usually responds well to antibiotics although more resistant cases occasionally require surgical draining.

Trigeminal Neuralgia/ Tic Douloureux

Trigeminal neuralgia is a fairly common condition that primarily affects older individuals. The pain is of a shooting or lightning type. It generally last only a few seconds but can recur on a repetitive basis.

Frequently when some portion of the face or mouth is stimulated (a trigger zone), the pain is confined to one side and is usually below the eye, although the forehead can be affected as well.

This malady is caused by irritation of the nerve fibers near the base of the brain. Occasionally, tumors of this nerve or compressive lesions of the surrounding tissue cause this type of problem.

The pain is described as unbearable and can lead to total disruption of the sufferer's lifestyle. Fortunately, trigeminal neuralgia usually responds to the medication Tegretol, although occasionally it is necessary to destroy nerve fibers via a surgical procedure.

Occipital Neuralgia

This is a common disorder that is often missed by family practitioners and neurologists alike. Great controversy surrounds the frequency or even the existence of this disorder. We have found the condition associated with neck trauma in persons injured in automobile accidents. While the pain can be similar to the shooting discomfort of trigeminal neuralgia, it is typically more of an aching pain radiating into the eye socket. Often the person also feels nausea.

This condition typically responds to oral anti-inflammatory medications or local injections, although sometimes destruction of the nerve is necessary.

Eye Disease

We have rarely seen eye problems as a cause for headache, although certainly one exception would be glaucoma, in which the pressure of the eyeball suddenly increases. With this disorder, there is extreme pain in the eye and in the forehead, and vomiting may occur. Usually the white portion of the eye is very red. This condition is an emergency that must be dealt with by an ophthalmologist as soon as possible to avoid blindness.

Pseudotumor Cerebri

The brain and the spinal cord are surrounded by fluid that forms at the base of the brain and travels through various channels. Eventually this fluid is resorbed close to the large superficial veins near the inner portion of the skull. This fluid not only provides a hydrostatic "cushion," but it also is important to the nutritional status of the brain itself—a sort of brain food.

Generally, the pressure in the system remains fairly constant, but if the pressure of this cerebrospinal fluid is extremely high, then the blood flow to the brain will be stopped and death will occur rapidly.

Headaches can occur with cerebrospinal pressure that is too low or too high. Mild to moderate elevations of pressure inside the bony skull are seen in the condition known as pseudotumor cerebri. As the name implies, the clinical picture resembles that of a brain tumor, and in the past, exploratory surgery was performed on individuals presenting with this clinical picture.

The common symptoms are headaches occasionally associated with nausea and vague visual symptoms. This condition is more common in women, especially in women who are overweight. It may also be seen in people taking some medications such as antibiotics and vitamins.

Therapy involves medication and sometimes also requires a series of lumbar punctures or even surgery.

Cluster Headaches

The cluster headache is a fairly common headache, which is usually associated with pain in the forehead and eye area and generally lasts no more than an hour. The cluster head pain is often linked with watering of the eye on the same side as the pain, as well as with a runny nose. Sometimes the eye droops and the pupil on the painful side becomes small.

The patient may have several attacks on one day and these headaches may occur regularly. Individuals who suffer from regular cluster headaches may have very coarse skin about the face.

Cluster headaches respond fairly well to medication, particularly high-dose oxygen.

One variation of the cluster headache is chronic paroxysmal hemicrania. This type of headache is similar to cluster headaches, although it more frequently occurs in middle-aged women and usually lasts for ten to twenty minutes. Such headaches may occur up to twelve times a day. Patients respond well to indomethacin (Indocin).

Temporal Arteritis (Giant Cell Arteritis)

Temporal arteritis, which primarily affects older individuals, is one of the more serious headaches and requires prompt evaluation and treatment.

The headache is usually described as a throbbing pain that is localized in the temporal area. Patients feel tired and ill, with an overall loss of energy. They may also report local tenderness, and merely brushing the hair may hurt. One frightening symptom is a sudden loss of vision in one eye. If this is neglected, vision can be severely impaired.

To diagnose this illness, a simple blood test, erythrocyte sedimentation rate (ESR) is often performed. This somewhat foreboding-sounding term refers merely to the rate at which red blood cells settle in a glass cylinder over a one-hour period. When giant cell arteritis is present, the ESR is usually several times the normal level.

In suspected cases of this disorder, an oral steroid is immediately prescribed, while preparations are made to remove a portion of the superficial temporal artery that is located in the temporal region. Prolonged therapy with oral steroids is often necessary.

Tumor

A common motivator for headache patients to see a doctor is the fear that they suffer from a malignant brain tumor. Yet only a very small minority of headache sufferers actually have brain tumors.

Headaches associated with brain tumors are fairly non-specific. If the pain is made worse by coughing, sneezing, or straining, or if it is generally worse in the morning, tumor would be a major consideration.

Meningitis

Severe headache is an almost invariable feature of meningitis. What is meningitis? It is an inflammation of the brain covering that results from infection. While there may be a history of exposure to meningitis or a history of middle ear or other infection, often there is no such history.

Viruses and bacteria account for most cases of meningitis, although many microorganisms can cause meningitis. Viral meningitis is usually self-limiting while bacterial meningitis is frequently fatal.

If diagnosed and treated early, the patient usually recovers entirely, although there may be such complications as seizures, deafness, or mental disabilities. The diagnosis of meningitis is confirmed with a spinal tap. (See the chapter on medical tests for further information on this procedure.)

Abnormal Blood Vessels

Various abnormalities of blood vessels can cause headaches. Arteriovenous malformations (AVMs) are abnormal blood vessels which channel blood from the arterial to the venous side of the circulation. Generally no headache results from this abnormality unless there is a hemorrhage. A hemorrhage can be life-threatening or it can cause fairly mild symptoms.

Headaches due to abnormal blood vessels may occur repeatedly, and for this reason can be misdiagnosed as migraine. Patients with this type of abnormality frequently have seizures, which complicate their clinical course.

Ruptured aneurysms also can cause severe headaches. An aneurysm is a "bleb" or a bubble-like expansion of an artery. The abnormal arterial expansion leads to weakness of the blood vessel wall and a high risk of hemorrhage.

The resulting condition, subarachnoid hemorrhage, is typically a sudden and very severe headache, often described by the patient as the "worst headache of my life." It is a true medical emergency and CT scan, angiography, and often lumbar puncture are needed to diagnose this condition. Surgery is usually recommended.

Stroke

Stroke can be defined as the death of a portion of the brain resulting from a disrupted supply of blood. This can be based on a clogged artery or a hemorrhage (excessive, sudden bleeding). The arteries are frequently blocked by debris from the heart or carotid arteries, or by the ultimate progression of atherosclerosis.

In the non-hemorrhagic stroke, headache is fairly common although usually mild. As with migraine, stroke frequently causes visual changes and thus can lead to a faulty diagnosis.

Medications

In a patient troubled by headaches, a careful medication history is essential. For example, it is now well known that aspirin as well as many other medications can actually cause headaches. In addition, suddenly withdrawing medications may lead to "rebound headaches."

Commonly used medications that are associated with headaches include nitroglycerin, captopril, indomethacin, cimetidine, and verapamil.

Emergency Headaches

Certainly not every headache should lead you to rush off to your doctor. Some guidelines may help you determine when a medical investigation is a good idea.

A sudden change in the severity or type of headache, or the appearance of a new kind of headache in someone over the age of 50 should. give rise to some concern. Also, headaches associated with mental symptoms or neurologic symptoms such as a drooping eye, muscle weakness, or the loss of balance should be reported to your doctor.

Headaches associated with intense neck pain or fever and headaches associated with straining, lifting, coughing, or sneezing suggest a more ominous type of headache. You should see your physician if your headache falls into these categories.

4

Women and Migraines

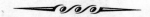

If you're a woman, your migraines may be caused by reactions to food, stress, or any of the other causes discussed in this book. Or your migraines may be directly connected to the fact that you are a woman. Or sometimes a combination of factors, such as eating a food trigger or experiencing severe stress, along with the onset of your period, is enough to thrust you into a migrainous state.

In the past, many physicians presumed that women with migraines were malingering (faking). They were also perceived as whiners—either stressed-out career women or bored housewives. Whatever the assumption, doctors often did not view a woman's migraines as a problem to be taken seriously.

Now, happily, most doctors *do* take women's migraines seriously. If your doctor does not, you should consider changing physicians (after you read chapter 8!).

Over two-thirds of all the people who suffer from migraines are female, and in many cases, the causes (or exacerbating factors) appear to be hormonal. Girls and boys have about the same incidence of migraine headaches, but after puberty, girls speed past boys in the migraine department.

What this means is that many women suffer from migraines premenstrually or just after their period starts. Sometimes the migraines go away during pregnancy, only to come back after the baby is born. (Just what you need: killer headaches along with the many hours of child care!)

Sometimes menopause means an end to migraines. And sometimes it means a beginning, if you are placed on estrogen replacement therapy (ERT) by your physician. Estrogen, whether you produce it in your body or it comes from a pill, can lead to migraine headaches.

Complicating it all, sometimes you may have a mild allergic reaction to food, stress, and so forth, or your body may have a slight reaction to medications. But when combined with menstruation or other hormonal changes, your brain pushes you over the edge into a full-fledged migraine. So you can't ignore the other probable causes of migraines described in other chapters. What you can do is try to isolate the causes and, when possible, eliminate them or mitigate them.

Therefore, we will cover the key female-related events that can cause or contribute to migraine headaches. We will also talk about some possible solutions that have worked in clinical trials and when individual doctors tried them on their patients.

It's great to be born female, but there's no reason, if you suffer from hormonally related migraines, why you should accept headache pain as your lot in life. Read this chapter and work with your physician, whether a gynecologist, primary care physician, neurologist, or other doctor, to resolve the problem—or at least reduce the instances and severity of your migraines.

Pre-Menstrual Syndrome and Migraines

A large proportion of women who do suffer from migraines (and who are still menstruating) report that their headaches occur a few days or just before the onset of menstruation. An estimated 60 percent of women with migraines report that their migraines can be directly correlated with the time before, during, or sometimes right after their periods.

Researchers believe that these migraines are related to fluctuating hormone levels, probably falling levels of estrogen. Many women have other physiological and even psychological effects, such as cramping and crankiness.

Your doctor has probably asked you to keep a headache diary, which will enable the two of you to identify possible causes and patterns in your headaches. You should also be sure to track your migraines in relation to your menstrual cycles. If headaches nearly always occur a few days before your period, then your migraines are probably hormone-related.

Many of the medications described elsewhere in this book, such as Imitrex, have proven very effective with women who suffer from migraines related to PMS.

Some physicians have also recommended preventive treatment for such migraineurs; for example, amitriptyline (Elavil) taken for a few days prior to when you think your cycle will start may provide some relief. Other physicians have found success with propranolol for that time frame just prior to the menses. (Yes, we know. You do have to be fairly "regular" to know when to start the medication.)

Other physicians have recommended percutaneous estradiol gel, both before and during the course of your menstrual period.

And still other physicians have recommended a low dose of estrogen for about one week before menstruation, in order to bring up decreasing levels of estrogen. Check with your physician to see what he or she recommends as the best strategy.

You should also avoid chocolate and caffeine premenstrually—no matter how much your body craves these substances! For many people, they are major migraine triggers.

Pregnancy May Bring Relief

In the majority of cases, when a woman becomes pregnant, her hormonal levels stabilize and those melancholy migraines go away—or at least become less agonizingly painful, especially in the first trimester of pregnancy. This is a good time since it's best to avoid most medications during pregnancy, particularly the early months. If you are pregnant, you should only take what is absolutely necessary to your health and the health of your child.

It's also a good idea to talk to your physician about your migraines while you are still pregnant, even though your suffering may be gone or minimal. Because those murderous migraines may come back, it's wise to have an attack plan. If possible, ask your physician to refer you to a good neurologist in your area.

Menopause

Large numbers of Baby Boomer women (born 1946–1964) are heading into menopause, and for many of them, this may mean, at long last, relief from migraines.

In many cases, however, physicians may decide that it would be a good idea for patients to take estrogen when they are menopausal, to avoid problems of osteoporosis (bone loss) and other symptoms of menopause. Be sure to notify your physician if you have suffered from migraines in the past and be double-sure to tell the doctor if your migraines seem to be related to taking birth control pills. Why? Because birth control pills are hormones, as is estrogen administered to menopausal women

Also, make sure that you really are in menopause before you agree to take estrogen. In one case, a woman's doctor decided that a thirty-something woman was probably in menopause because of various symptoms and also because she had had a subtotal hysterectomy in her late twenties.

Although she still had her ovaries, her doctor presumed they were no longer working so put her on estrogen.

For several years, the woman complained about severe headaches, and she continued to take frequent headache medications along with her estrogen. Finally, one day she read that estrogen could cause migraines and decided to stop taking it. The migraines went away. Then she started the estrogen again (at the urging of her doctor), and the migraines came back. She stopped the estrogen again and the migraines disappeared again.

The woman went to see another doctor, who also ardently believed in the benefits of estrogen replacement therapy, but the woman was skeptical. The doctor ordered a blood test to check the woman's hormonal levels, in part to prove to the woman that she needed the estrogen. The blood tests came back normal. This meant that the woman had never needed the estrogen, and was essentially overdosing her body with it.

The moral of this story is this: If you are under age fifty and still have ovaries, and if your doctor wants you to start taking estrogen, insist on a blood test of your hormonal levels first.

Medications Causing Migraines

Medications can greatly influence migraines as well, sometimes causing them to occur. For example, birth control pills can cause migraines, particularly during the period when you are off the pill. As previously mentioned, estrogen may also cause migraines, although this is certainly not always the case.

Birth Control Pills

If you are on birth control pills and are suffering from recurring migraines, you should probably consider an alternative method of avoiding pregnancy. The Pill is easy and efficient, and it's true most other methods of birth control are messy and annoying. But if you can get rid of your migraines, it's worth it to consider another method.

It's also important to note that it may take several months for the birth control pill to "clear" from your system, so you may not gain immediate relief from stopping the medication. Certainly do not expect that the day you stop taking the Pill is the day you can kiss your headaches good-bye forever.

Estrogen Replacement Therapy (ERT)

Women who are menopausal may suffer from migraines if they are placed on estrogen replacement therapy. Or they may find that their migraines go away!

If you took the Pill as a younger woman and had to stop because of migraines, it's possible that you may also suffer from migraines with ERT. But it is not inevitable! Our bodies change as we age, and since improved formulations are developed all the time, it is possible that changing the brand of ERT could resolve the problem for you.

A Combination of Causes

Although menstrual cycles and fluctuations of estrogen levels can cause migraines, the problem can also be caused by a variety of triggers. For example, if some foods are headache triggers for you, you should definitely avoid those foods before your period. To determine whether any foods trigger your headaches, track them with a headache diary (see Appendix for example).

If it's cheese that sets you off, be sure to avoid cheese premenstrually, because you don't need the combination of the food trigger and the hormonal fluctuation to signal your brain: "Time for a real doozy of a migraine!"

Medications That Work

Many of the medications described elsewhere in this book are very effective for women with hormonally related migraines. For example, in one trial of 669 menstruating women, all with migraines, it was determined that Sumatriptan worked far better than a placebo (sugar pill) in clearing up the migraine.

In fact, this medication apparently worked even better in women with menstrually related migraines as compared to women with non-menstrually related migraines. In addition, it provided continued relief for up to 24 hours for both groups of women.

In addition to such previously mentioned medications as Sansert, other medications are effective for menstrually associated migraines. Diuretics, commonly referred to as "water pills," are often helpful. Diamox is a unique type of water pill that is very effective when taken a few days prior to the onset of menstruation and then daily throughout the course of menstruation. This seems to be a most effective treatment for women who retain excessive water during their periods.

Migraine can behave differently in the two sexes. The cataclysmic hormonal changes that only women endure—such as pregnancy, contraception, and menstruation—can interact profoundly with migraine. Physicians can avoid many treatment failures by taking a careful history of the nature and cycle of a woman's headaches then tailoring the therapy to her specific needs.

5

Migraine in Children
and Adolescents

———◦◦◦———

We have already discussed different headache types, particularly migraine, in adults. However, because children and young adults with migraine differ slightly from standard sufferers of migraine headache disorders, we will now focus on the younger age groups.

Medical History Is
Critically Important

First of all, as in any good medical evaluation, the history is everything. One difficulty of treating children with migraine is obtaining a clear, concise, and accurate history. A child may not be able to describe his headaches and may not be able to characterize them or to explain their frequency, intensity, or severity.

In addition, a child may not have the language or the skills needed to describe the different components of the headache as most adults can. Therefore, it is crucial to have a clear history obtained not only from the child, but from other observers, particularly parents, siblings, and oftentimes teachers. Even school peers may add historical perspective, which can be extremely helpful in completing the puzzle that makes up pediatric and adolescent migraine.

Use a Headache Diary

As with other types of migraine and headache disorders, it is important to keep a headache diary, to determine if there are environmental, social, psychological, physical, chemical, or food triggers. (A headache diary sample is provided in the Appendix.)

Rule Out Serious Problems

Also, it is important to rule out serious or dangerous types of headache symptoms. Headaches that warrant immediate attention in the pediatric population would include the following:

- Headaches that are progressive in severity or intensity
- Headaches that are associated with weakness or clumsiness
- Headaches that are associated with a stiff neck or fever
- Any type of head tilt, head bob, or gait clumsiness
- A child with a chronic illness who develops headache
- Headache associated with a large head
- Children with chronic infections, particularly of the ears, teeth, or mouth

Categorize the Headache

Barring a serious organic or structural illness, headache disorders in children should be classified into either migraine type headaches or muscle type headaches.

While the characteristics are not absolute, frequently children suffering from a migraine headache disorder will describe a throbbing, hemicranial (one-half of the skull or head), periodic, sick headache.

In contrast, those children and young adults suffering from muscle contraction headaches will often describe a severe pulling, stretching, or tearing type pain, often at the base of the skull. Often, the child will describe the headache as being located everywhere over the scalp and head, not in just one isolated place.

The headaches that are muscle contraction in origin are often daily, chronic, and last for a significant period of time. There are rarely any associated neurologic, motor, or sensory deficits, or any associated nausea.

"Runs in the Family"

Children with migraine disorders will often have a strong family history of migraine, as do adult sufferers. The migraine may awaken the child from sleep, and may be associated with a warning or aura, as we described earlier with many adults. Muscle contraction headaches are often lacking these characteristics. In addition, children with migraine disorders often will respond to traditional migraine medications, while those with muscle contraction headaches will rarely respond to migraine medications.

Sleep Can Help

As we were taught during a neurology training program, and which has become an invaluable lesson throughout our practice, children who suffer from a migraine headache disorder often have "sick headaches." Frequently, the best therapy is sleep, and parents will often respond to the question "What makes the headache better?" with an unequivocal "Sleep!" If children experiencing migraines can just get to sleep, when they wake up, they're often fine.

Children also have an incomplete form of migraines, experiencing the nausea, the acute vomiting, and the extreme fatigue frequently associated in adults as the post-migraine chemical depletion. After a period of sleep, the neurochemicals of the brain seem to be restored, and the children have their routine energy once again.

Common or Classic?

Children with migraine can often have all forms of migraine, including common migraine without a warning or aura. They can also have "classic migraine," which often begins with the visual disturbance, described frequently as flashes of lights, zigzag lines, jagged lights, and patterns of light distortions.

Many times we find that instead of having children describe the pattern of lights and the disturbance to us, if we ask them to simply draw the pattern of disturbance, we can get clear and precise details with regard to their migraine warning.

Of possible concern is a child who presents with a complicated migraine. These children can have the full spectrum of migraine illness, as well as complications such as weakness, numbness, and clumsiness, which often mimic a stroke-like syndrome. Any time a child presents with a complicated migraine, neurologic evaluation is absolutely necessary.

Confusional States

We should make one brief comment regarding a variant of migraine headache—the headache disturbance that presents predominantly as a confusional state. Oftentimes, children with periodic confusional episodes will have a diagnosis of seizures, of daydreaming or staring spells, or of hypo-glycemia.

Actually, migraine can present in any form, and in young children, it does rarely present as a confusion and disorientation syndrome. However, we find that this is a diagnosis that is made only after other more serious diagnoses have been excluded. Diagnostic testing, such as MRI or CAT scan of the brain, brain wave scan, and often, lumbar puncture, is usually necessary to exclude other more serious illnesses.

Migraine with Seizure Disorder

In addition, a small percentage of individuals have migraines connected with seizure disorder. Children who suffer from migraine headaches often have abnormalities on the brain wave scan during the headache disorder, which then become normal between headache episodes.

It can be quite complicated to differentiate between a seizure event that is not accompanied by involuntary movements and a migraine headache disorder that is accompanied with altered blood flow in the brain, producing abnormal brain wave changes.

Other Symptoms

Although children may have the headache pain without associated symptoms, a majority will also have the nausea, vomiting, stomach cramping, and abdominal discomfort that adults often suffer when they experience migraine attacks.

Just as in migraines affecting adults, in a pediatric migraine, the stomach wall activity slows down during the acute migraine attack. For that reason, many medications are indeed ineffective. Therefore, often we must resort to using medications that are not given by mouth, but rather by rectal suppository or even by injection.

Precipitating Triggers for Children and Adolescents

While we have described different types of headache symptoms in children in the previous paragraphs, it is important to realize that, in addition to the standard migraine triggers, there are many other precipitating factors in the child population.

Often, psychological factors, such as change in school environment, as well as physiological factors, including change in hormone level, onset of menarche, and dehydration, play a role in triggering migraines. Children are also extremely sensitive to fluctuations in routine, particularly to missed meals, as well as hypoglycemic events. This is a frequent cause of headache syndrome.

By asking children to chart their migraine attacks, we can often identify certain foods that act as triggers. It seems simple enough to eliminate these foods from the diet; however, as many parents know, gaining complete cooperation from a child or adolescent is often difficult. For this reason, making reasonable compromises with diet modifications is often best for migraine prevention.

Sleep Problems

If the patient suffers from headaches related to a disordered sleep cycle, such as insomnia, multiple awakenings from sleep at night, or terminal insomnia (waking up too early), we find that pharmacologic as well as non-prescription sleep aids are often effective.

We have had a great deal of success using small doses of Ambien, a relatively new sleep medication. Of course, body height and weight measurements are absolutely necessary to determine the safety of any prescription medication.

Nevertheless, we find that when we can readjust the sleep cycle, not only is it beneficial for the migraine management, it often seems to provide increased energy and alertness during the daytime, which produces a positive effect in school performance. This seems to have a snowball effect, producing positive self-esteem and ultimately leading into decreased stress, anxiety, and a reduction in headache frequency.

Treatments

We try to avoid significant centrally acting medications in our practice, as these will often cause clouding of consciousness, confusion, and decreased memory and attention, which can negatively impact on school performance.

Rather, as with the adult population, non-pharmacologic treatments are often pursued first. We have found biofeedback, guided imagery, and relaxation techniques helpful in allowing children to control their own headache syndrome. This, of course, works better with older children and adolescents.

Headaches can also be an outward manifestation or cry for attention, particularly with depressed children. Since lifestyle changes and self-image issues may be triggering the headaches, counseling or supportive therapy that leads to helping the child develop adequate and appropriate coping mechanisms is often more effective in reducing the headache severity and frequency in the long term, rather than medication management in the short-term.

On rare occasions, we do use antidepressant medication, not only for the antidepressant effect, but also for its effect on the central nervous system chemicals, as described in other chapters. Particularly, medications with amitriptyline, nortriptyline, and serotonin seem somewhat more effective compared to other medications for depression and relief of headache pain.

Medications

When we do use prescription medications, we try to target the type of headache, the nature of the headache with regard to daytime vs. nighttime, and the associated symptoms that occur with each headache episode. For example, the children who experience confusion, dizziness, disorientation, and have positive brain wave scans are often best treated with medications such as phenobarbital, rarely with Dilantin or Tegretol. All three of these medications are also quite effective as anti-seizure medication.

A common medication for headache therapy and pain relief is cyproheptadine (Periactin), given two to three times per day in one-half to one 4 mg tablet, depending on the child's age and body weight. A beta-blocker (Inderal), a cornerstone of migraine management, is also very helpful.

We usually delay prescribing this medication until the child shows us a series of headaches, particularly more than two in any one given month. This is used predominantly for prophylactic (preventive) management, and it is not quite as effective for management of the acute migraine attack.

True pain medications, as we have discussed earlier, such as combination medications (aspirin, phenacetin, codeine, fiorinal #3) are often helpful for pain management. The side effect of these medications is that they do cause drowsiness, as do some of the barbiturate medications, and therefore the child will need to rest, avoid exertional activity, and avoid activities which require focused concentration.

These types of medications are habit-forming and possibly addicting. Medication by rectum, such as Phenergan rectal suppositories, are often quite effective for the nausea, as well as for sedation, which can be an effective therapy in and of itself, as noted previously.

Other medication, such as Cafergot, can also be given by rectal suppository or by mouth. Again, if the headache has been present more than 30 to 60 minutes, medications given by mouth often lose their effectiveness, and do not produce any of the desired effects—pain relief, sleep initiation, and muscle contraction relief.

Conclusion

It is important to realize that no one treatment fits every individual; therefore, obtaining the history of each child is absolutely essential. Maintaining a careful headache diary, avoiding food triggers, and identifying and eliminating external and social triggers are extremely important, possibly even more so than in the adult population.

If a child with recurrent headaches fails to improve with the previously listed measures, a consultation with a pediatric neurologist or neurologist specializing in headache management is often necessary to help fine-tune treatment regimens.

6

Non-Food Migraine Triggers

⤚⤙⤚⤙

W e've emphasized the critical importance of your physician taking a good headache history to enable effective
treatment of your migraines. In the initial interview with you,
as well as during your subsequent visits, the doctor must
work hard to identify the primary factors leading to your
headache problem. Once the identification of a trigger is
made, you have an excellent chance of improvement with an
effective, safe, and inexpensive therapy.

What's a Trigger?

A trigger is a factor, either internal or external, which can pro-
voke a migraine attack. The trigger is not the cause of the
headache, but acts instead as a catalyst that sets in motion
the complex chain of events culminating in a migraine attack.
A trigger can be external stimuli, such as bright light,
certain foods, or weather changes, to name just a few. Or a

trigger could come from within, such as hunger, fatigue, or stress.

If trigger factors can be identified and subsequently avoided or minimized, then you will be saved from the prospect of medications or non-pharmacological treatments that could have side effects, cost big bucks, and have unpredictable effects.

More than half of all migraine sufferers will, with effort, be able to identify the trigger mechanism that is uniquely their own. But it is also true that susceptibility to triggers can vary even in the same person. For example, women may be more susceptible to triggers during the postmenstrual or premenstrual period than at other times during their menstrual cycle.

Age can also affect susceptibility to a trigger factor. Alcohol consumption is one good example of this phenomenon. Some people with a migrainous tendency are able to tolerate even large quantities of alcohol at a younger age, but later in life may find that even one drink of an alcoholic beverage can bring on an agonizing migraine attack.

It is also true that some triggers affect the sexes unequally. For example, one study revealed that weather changes, missing a meal, and the odor of perfume or cigarette smoke were much more common triggers of migraine in women than in men, while sexual activity seemed to trigger migraines more commonly in males.

Common Triggers

Stress heads the list of all psychological triggers and also may be the most potent trigger of migraine in general. Some experts believe that more than 50 percent of all migraines are triggered by some type of emotionally stressful situation. And not only are migraines more frequent and severe during times of great stress, but the other bad news is that they tend to last for a longer period of time.

Many people who suffer from migraines identify the onset of the disorder in their lives as directly associated with a time of severe stress. Stress may be financial, academic, marital, or of some other nature.

In younger people, migraines triggered by stress may be associated with worrying about such things as examinations or plans to attend (or perform in) an important concert or recital. Sometimes the migraines that occur in these cases happen before the event and sometimes afterward.

Sometimes patients find their migraines cluster in weekends, which seems particularly unfair after a week of hard work. Possible reasons for this could be changes in sleep patterns, consumption of caffeine-containing beverages (more or less), alcohol use, smoking, or other factors.

Case History

A 45-year-old woman with a 20-year history of migraine was seen in our neurologic clinic. She was required to attend three to four major fashion events each year. Before each show, the patient experienced several weeks of intense activity related to preparing for the show. She sustained a very high level of activity until the end of the fashion show. Then, invariably, the patient developed a migraine attack that lasted three to four days.

Recognizing the stress of the fashion show planning as her trigger, we prescribed preventive medication as well as ergotamine, which proved ineffective in helping this patient. However, self-administered Imitrex has proven very effective in managing this woman's headaches, especially their intensity. Having access to rapid and effective treatment greatly increased her self-confidence as well.

Many Different Medications May Trigger Migraines

Sometimes a medication that you are taking to resolve another medical problem is your migraine trigger. Medications used to control high blood pressure, arthritis, estrogen replacement therapy (ERT), antibiotics, and even medications to relieve chest pain have all been implicated in causing headaches in susceptible people. In fact, many of these medications can cause headaches in people who are not usually prone to migraines.

Nitroglycerin is a good example of a medication that can trigger typical migraine headaches. While this medication can also cause headaches in non-migraineurs, it can lead to devastating migraines in susceptible people within minutes.

Indomethacin and other nonsteroidal/anti-inflammatory drugs (NSAIDS) can be effective in aiding the migraineur and can also cause an intense headache associated with an inflammatory response in the brain membranes. Withdrawal from this medication can cause an intense headache.

Illegal drugs are also associated with migraines. Heroin and cocaine use can cause headaches and migraines. Some people have become addicted to cocaine as a result of this drug's effect on the migraine. Such headaches can occur immediately after use or within the withdrawal phases.

Sleep

Many migraineurs report that inducing sleep is the most effective means of aborting a migraine attack, insisting that their migraine will not relent until they are allowed to sleep.

But besides being therapeutic in the treatment of migraine, an alteration in the sleeping pattern can be a potent migraine trigger in some people, possibly affecting women more than men.

Oversleeping can often cause migraine. So if you get up every day at 6:00 A.M., it's not such a great idea to sleep until noon on the weekend. In addition, shift work and jet lag should be avoided by susceptible people whenever possible. Of course, generating a "sleep debt," that is, going for long periods of time with less sleep than your body actually needs, may also be a powerful trigger.

Exercise

We frequently emphasize the value of exercise in this book because exercise can have a therapeutic effect on migraine. Yet it can also exacerbate a migraine attack, especially when the person is unaccustomed to a particular exercise. This problem seems to be more commonly associated with such intense activity as running and racquet sports, and tends to affect the sexes equally.

Many different factors that can contribute to the exercise-related migraine include climactic conditions and altitude as well as the hydration and nutritional state of the exercising person. Also, the changing heart rate, pulse, and breathing patterns associated with exercise can all play some role as migraine triggers.

Sexual Activity

Men whose migraines are triggered by sex find they occur near the point of orgasmic release. Such headaches are often indistinguishable from a typical migraine attack. Clearly such a headache can be very distressing. Not only that, but this kind of headache is often resistant to medications and thus can have devastating consequences for the individual.

Another sexually related headache is the benign sex headache, which, again, affects men more often than women. This type of headache also occurs right at the time of climax, but has no clear relationship to the migraine headache.

On the other hand, orgasm may also relieve the migraine in some people. One woman reported she was able to partially control her migraines through masturbation.

Smoking

Tobacco use can be a potent migraine trigger for some people. This appears to be more true for women than for men. There may be many reasons for this—tobacco increases carbon dioxide, decreases oxygen delivery to the brain, and actually acts as a direct toxin in some cases.

Hunger

Missing a meal can be a powerful migraine trigger in some migraineurs and also appears to be a problem more often for women than for men. In one study, missing a meal was a triggering mechanism in up to 40 percent of those suffering from migraine. It is possible that the mechanism for hunger as a trigger for migraine could be hypoglycemia, although there is little support in the literature for this theory.

Hypoglycemia can certainly cause migraines in some people and is often caused by the person eating a meal high in simple sugars. Shortly after eating such a meal, the blood sugar tends to rise, only to fall to a fairly low level several hours later. Avoid such meals if this is a problem for you.

Weather Changes

Many people report a migraine during a sudden change in barometric pressure, such as occurs prior to a thunderstorm. Women seem more susceptible to weather changes than are men. With drops in barometric pressure, joint capsules (such as in the jaw, hand/finger joints, and so on.) will swell. If there is any tendency for the joints to be inflamed (as in TMJ), this swelling will lead to pain and possibly trigger a migraine.

Sight and Sound

An estimated one-third of all migraine sufferers find that glaring sunlight is a triggering mechanism for their migraines, although how or why this happens is unclear. As a result, many migraineurs avoid exposure to bright sunlight, such as snow skiing, water outings, or trips to the beach or other situations. People with this problem may wear sunglasses virtually all the time that they are outdoors. Another related trigger is irregular illumination, such as fluorescent light bulbs, computer monitors, or strobe lights generate.

In some people, loud noises from heavy machinery, loud music, automobile horns, and such can trigger a migraine.

Odor

Certain smells can be strong trigger mechanisms for some people. This problem can be incapacitating when the sufferer is unable to eliminate these odors from the immediate environment. Odors that cause problems in susceptible individuals often emanate from gasoline and cleaning solutions, as well as perfumes, lotions, and deodorants.

Every effort should be made to identify the offending agent, and family members and others should be enlisted to help get rid of them. Individuals whose migraines are triggered by odors can be virtually powerless in many social settings.

Spinal Disorders

Over recent years, the medical profession has become increasingly aware of the tendency of spine disorders to trigger migraines. This is particularly true for neck disorders, but recent publications also suggest that back pain can contribute to headaches.

Osteoarthritis (the wear-and-tear arthritis) of the neck, as well as chronic muscle irritation related to injury or chronic tension, can trigger migraine attacks in susceptible people. In addition, neck injuries are often causes of increased frequency, duration, and severity of headaches in individuals who suffered from migraines prior to the accident.

In one study of patients with chronic low back pain, the researcher found that 60 percent of the patients also reported headaches. Only half of them had reported headaches prior to the onset of their low back pain. These headaches were not only muscle tension type but also migraine.

We have seen several individuals of both sexes in whom an exacerbation of the chronic low back syndrome was also accompanied by a severe attack of migraine headache. In the Appendix, we outline a series of neck exercises, as well as list many daily activities that, when performed properly, can help reduce these types of triggers.

Case History

A 28-year-old woman came to our neurologic clinic for evaluation of head and neck pain. The patient reported a ten-year history of migraines that were primarily left-sided and associated with photophobia, nausea, vomiting, and general malaise lasting up to 24 hours. Prior to a "whiplash injury" in a car accident, the patient had two to three headaches per year. After the accident, she reported daily headaches.

The patient was enrolled in a twelve-week cervical reconditioning program comprised of a rigorous daily stretching exercise as well as a biweekly strengthening program. During the course of the twelve-week regimen, the patient's neck pain improved, as did her daily headaches. The frequency of her migraine attacks has reverted to the pre-injury level.

Allergy and Migraine

The presumed connection between migraine and allergy is certainly not new. For over a hundred years, debate has raged on over what the actual role of allergic reaction is in producing a migraine headache.

While most neurologists do not feel that an allergic reaction is a potent migraine generator, the concept still has staunch advocates, including the support of public opinion. We hear at least several times a month from patients who are convinced that they suffer from migraines as a direct result of allergy. Part of this misconception is the patient's inaccurate definition of migraine. It is true, however, that allergies can certainly cause headaches. For that reason, we will discuss the nature of an allergic reaction and explore the basis for allergy as a legitimate trigger of migraine.

What Is an Allergic Reaction Anyway?

The word allergy is a composite of allos (other) and ergon (action), implying some type of mobilization against foreign chemicals. The "allergen" is the chemical toward which the allergic reaction is directed.

After an organism is exposed to an allergen (sensitized), then arsenals of chemicals (antibodies) can be produced by the body to react with the invading allergen. When the added allergen and the antibody unite, a kind of biological hell breaks out. Different types of cells are immediately summoned to the war zone. Potent chemicals are produced and released near the site of the first skirmish.

The result is essentially an inflammatory response with the attendant swelling, increased blood flow, heat production, and often, pain. If this reaction occurs in your nasal membranes (rhinitis), there will be increased production of secretions (runny nose), sneezing, and various degrees of narrowing of the nasal passages. If this occurs in your airways (asthma), the typical wheezing of the asthmatic is observed and some degree of narrowing of the air passages can occur. Occasionally this can be fatal.

It should also be noted that allergens do not have to be foreign substances, but can be part of your body; for example, some diseases cause the body to begin forming antibodies to its own tissues. An example of this would include some types of arthritis, lupus, and possibly even diabetes.

How Does Allergy Relate to Migraine?

Early (and continued) contentions that migraine and allergy were inevitably and inextricably connected were not based on any formal research but were merely the project of unschooled speculation. Now we do have some documented evidence of a weak link.

In the first half of this century, there were frequent reports of patients who were allergic to various foods. The reported patients had some type of allergic skin response to a specific type of food, but these claims were not substantiated by formal, case-controlled studies.

In addition, there was at least one report of a patient who developed a migraine when given a food type to which he had a demonstrated allergy. However, it was later demonstrated that when that same patient was not aware that he was consuming the alleged allergen, no headache would occur.

Another major problem with this type of research is that patients frequently will have a positive skin allergic response and have no type of demonstrable allergic symptoms and also no migraine. The more modern serologic studies aren't much better.

A fairly convincing evidence for a connection between food, allergy, and migraine was published in 1985. In this study, patients who had allergies to various foodstuffs, including wheat, corn, egg, and so on, were tested with food challenge (served a meal containing the suspected allergen). These patients were found to develop a headache within thirty minutes of ingesting the offending food item, even when they were unaware they had consumed it.

Some of these patients were demonstrated to have increased levels of histamine (an important chemical released during an immune response) in their blood after eating the food.

A more recently published study demonstrates correlation between food allergy and migraine. This study focused on children, age seven to eighteen, suffering from migraine. The children were divided into two groups: those who continued their customary diet, and those placed on a hypoallergenic regimen, which included only eight very simple foods for a duration of four weeks.

The control group demonstrated no change in their headache pattern, while the diet-restricted individuals improved. Fifty percent of the diet-restricted group found their headaches were entirely eliminated, while most of the others reported a significant improvement in the pattern of the headaches. The most common offending food types in this study were cacao (chocolate), banana, egg, and hazelnuts.

The Histamine Connection

Histamine is discussed in this context because of its role in the mediation of the allergic response. Interestingly, histamine can cause dilation of the blood vessels in the scalp, which is seen in migraine, and can also cause severe, throbbing headaches, even in patients without migraine.

Typically, patients with migraine will get a headache from a smaller dose of histamine than is needed to generate a headache in a non-migraineur. In addition, the headache usually is experienced on the side where the migraine usually occurs. This so-called histamine headache can be entirely blocked by medications that block the effect of histamine, while these same medications have no effect whatsoever on a genuine migraine attack.

Some German authors believe that migraine is caused by histamine, but not on the basis of allergy. They feel that the histamine in the diet leads to a migraine attack. For this reason, they have proposed a regimen for elimination of histamine from the diet.

The investigators developed a diet in which fish, cheese, sausage, pickled cabbage, wine, and beer were excluded for four weeks. The authors report a major reduction in the frequency of headaches on the elimination diet. They furthermore postulate that the basic biochemical defect in the patient is actually a deficiency of the enzyme involved in the biochemical elimination of histamine. We find this an interesting theory, but certainly one that will need further investigation.

Other Types of Allergy in Migraine

Population studies have been attempted to demonstrate a link between migraine and atopic (allergic) diseases, such as hives, asthma, and rhinitis. Both migraine and these allergic illnesses frequently occur in the same individual. But studies have not been able to demonstrate a clearly increased frequency of these two disorders in specific individuals.

The largest association was with rhinitis, and the authors report that rhinitis is particularly common in children whose mothers suffer from migraine. At this point, we feel there is much conflicting information with regard to the coexistence of these two disorders in the same patient and await a more definitive resolution of this matter.

Back in 1955, an interesting study demonstrated that migraine headaches can be a consequence of allergic illness. Twenty-eight patients were studied, all of whom had migraines, as well as rhinitis or asthma. The specific allergens to which the patient was known to be allergic were injected into the patient, thus reproducing the allergic symptoms. In most patients receiving the injections, a typical migraine occurred.

It should also be mentioned at this point that people with these types of allergic illnesses also have other problems that can increase the frequency of their headaches in general, and more specifically, their migraines. For example, these patients are often depressed and stressed because of their illness.

It should be noted that medications to block the action of histamines—including steroids, decongestants, and theophylline—can also affect the frequency and severity of headaches in people who are prone to attacks.

By being aware of possible triggers, you and your doctor can engage in a broad, open-minded search for the offending factor. The ideal outcome of any encounter with your physician is to eliminate your problem without drugs, surgery, radiation, or other potentially hazardous therapy. With migraine, this is often possible.

7

Food Fright

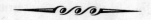

That migraines can be provoked by dietary influences is a fact that the lay public readily accepts. Many migraine sufferers have one or more foods they avoid.

The prospect of specifically identifying a chemical trigger in dietary migraine is a complex task. It should be remembered that triggers are facilitatory mechanisms that can lead to a full-blown migraine attack, only if various unknown other preconditions are met. For example, a long-awaited deadline may come and go without provoking a migraine attack in a woman whose menstrual cycle did not coincide with the deadline in question.

Similarly, a migraineur may imbibe large quantities of nitrite-containing foods or large amounts of red wine with relative impunity—unless the other factors involved in the migraine-producing process are also at work. Since response to a trigger varies even in a specific individual, it is difficult to research and form conclusions about this matter.

Furthermore, if a migraineur firmly believes that a specific food product will bring on a migraine attack, this is likely to occur as a self-fulfilling prophecy. Often, if the same patient is given the same food unknowingly, the migrainous response will not occur as predictably. Moreover, there may be a dose response for the triggering mechanism. Small amounts of the offending agents may be taken without provoking an attack. Even more perplexing is the fact that ingestion of the migraine-provoking agent may be related to a migraine attack already in progress, as is suggested with chocolate.

Food Triggers

Although much of the data presented in the literature on the subject of diet and migraine is anecdotal and based on questionable scientific rigor, we have concluded that there are potent triggers in the dietary sphere. As we have stated elsewhere in this work, the more systematic and open-minded the search for a trigger is, the more likely the individual is to succeed in identifying and eliminating migraine-provoking factors.

Alcohol

Alcohol is one of the most frequently identified dietary triggers by migraineurs. Interestingly, there is little documentation of alcohol per se as being the actual trigger. The studies to date suggest that the triggers are actually the various other components of alcoholic beverages that trigger a migraine in susceptible individuals.

Purer alcoholic beverages such as vodka, gin, and white wine seem to be tolerated fairly well by migraineurs while red wine is thought to be much more potent in terms of migraine stimulation. The chemical tyramine (vide infra) has been touted as being the offending agent in red wine. This has not been proven with any degree of certainty, but the observation that red wine is a more potent trigger is fairly commonly accepted.

Sugar Substitutes

Headache is a frequently reported side effect of the artificial sweetener aspartame (NutraSweet). This ingredient is used in diet sodas, as well as in a wide range of other products. The scientific data at hand are conflicting with regard to aspartame's role in provoking headaches. While this substance may not be a very frequent trigger of actual migraine headaches, it should be regarded as being suspect until further data exonerate this additive.

Caffeine

Caffeine is a ubiquitous substance in most countries of the world. It is abundant in coffee seeds and tea leaves, as well as in cocoa. In the American society, most caffeine is ingested through coffee drinking. Other sources would include tea, cocoa, and chocolate. Caffeine is also added to various over-the-counter pain relievers such as Anacin, and is also present in most soft drinks.

The role of caffeine in triggering migraine is probably not related to the immediate ingestion of this compound but rather to its withdrawal. Continued caffeine ingestion can be addictive, similar to nicotine, cocaine, heroin, and so on. The typical withdrawal picture includes headache, lassitude, restlessness, and even confusion.

Typical headaches undistinguished from typical migraine can be triggered by this withdrawal state in individuals suffering from migraine. Often, a cup of coffee will relieve headache symptoms. The withdrawal headaches usually occur by 16 hours after the last cup of coffee. It is not uncommon for the weekend to be a setting for caffeine withdrawal, as many individuals drink large amounts of caffeine during the work week and more modest amounts during the weekend.

Sodium Nitrite

Many preserved foods, including meat and fish, contain the preservative sodium nitrite. This substance, which is usually found in prepared meats such as bologna, sausage, hot dogs, and bacon, can cause severe throbbing headaches in individuals not suffering from migraine. They can also produce headaches undistinguished from a migraine in individuals suffering from this condition.

Many migraineurs avoid food products containing sodium nitrite since they can trigger headaches. It is the practice in our Headache Clinic to recommend avoidance of nitrite-containing products.

Citrus Fruits

Citrus fruits are universally touted as being among the most healthful features of any diet. However, citrus can be a potent trigger for migraines in susceptible individuals. It is thought that some of the nitrogen-containing substances in citrus have an effect on blood vessels and are capable of leading to a migraine attack.

While it would appear a bit extreme for migraineurs to avoid citrus altogether, careful analysis of the dietary diary should be undertaken to establish a possible role of citrus fruits in migraine provocation.

Monosodium Glutamate

Monosodium glutamate (MSG) is another chemical prevalent in Western diets. It is used as an additive to amplify the taste of various types of food. The consumer faces the difficult task of establishing the presence of MSG in many types of foods because euphemistic and confusing terms (such as "hydrolyzed protein" and "natural flavorings") are often used without specifically identifying the MSG content in a given product.

While MSG is inextricably associated in the popular mind with Chinese food, it is present in a wide range of food, including frozen dinners, potato chips, salad dressings, various seasoning products, and fast food such as fried chicken and hamburgers.

If MSG is ingested in sufficient amounts, it will produce a reaction that might include lightheadedness, abdominal pain, nausea, oral and facial numbness, headache, and chest pain within 30 minutes of the intake. This is popularly called the "Chinese restaurant syndrome."

Migraineurs frequently reported developing a typical migraine attack after eating even minute doses of MSG. It is the general practice of our Headache Clinic to advise patients to avoid foods containing this particular compound.

Tyramine

Tyramine belongs to a number of nitrogen-containing chemicals that directly or indirectly affect the caliber of blood vessels, thereby influencing blood pressure and the function of various organ systems. The effects of tyramine are similar to that of adrenaline and other related nitrogen-containing, physiologically active compounds.

After eating foods high in tyramine content, the migraineur may experience a typical attack within hours. The literature is rife with conflicting data regarding the importance of tyramine as a migraine trigger. In our view, it is a potent trigger in selected individuals, particularly if it is ingested in large amounts.

High tyramine-containing foodstuffs would include aged cheeses such as Brie, Roquefort, and Camembert. Many. processed meats including bologna and salami contain large amounts of tyramine, as do sauerkraut and some beverages, such as beer and various wines. Migraineurs should be aware that many other foods have low levels of tyramine until spoilage. Improperly stored fish and liver can accumulate large amounts of tyramine over a fairly short period of time.

While the actual prevalence of tyramine-sensitive migraineurs is unclear, we recommend that patients in our Headache Clinic avoid large amounts of tyramine and we deliver instructions for elimination of these foodstuffs.

Other nitrogen-containing compounds with similar effects would include phenylethylamine, which may be the primary trigger in those individuals sensitive to chocolate. We think that there is good evidence supporting the concept of dietary factors as potent triggers for migraines in selected individuals. And yet we also believe that the influence placed on dietary migraine by many physicians, including some neurologists, is excessive.

Instead, we believe that a systematic approach—that is, a consistent and accurate dietary diary—is a more rational approach to dietary modification and will obviate indiscriminate banning of potentially nutritious and pleasurable classes of foodstuffs, rendering the migraineur a "dietary invalid."

Diet and Headache

According to the National Headache Foundation, the following foods may trigger migraine headaches:

Food that has been fermented, marinated, or pickled

Foods containing MSG

Sausage, bologna, pepperoni, salami, summer sausage, hot dogs

Chicken livers, paté

Herring, pickled or dried

Ripened cheeses such as Cheddar, Emmentaler, Stilton, Brie, Camembert

(Permissible cheese includes American cheese, cottage cheese, cream cheese, and Velveeta.)

Sour cream (more than ½ cup per day)

Nuts, peanut butter

Sourdough bread

Crackers or breads containing either cheese or chocolate

Broad beans, lima beans, fava beans, and snow peas

Figs, raisins, papayas, avocados, red plums (more than ½ cup per day)

Citrus fruits (more than ½ cup per day)

Bananas (more than ½ per day)

Chocolate

Pizza

Tea, coffee, or cola (more than 2 cups per day)

Alcoholic beverages (If you decide to drink, limit to two normal-sized drinks of Haute Sauterne, Riesling, Seagram's VO, or Cutty Sark.)

8

Choosing the Right Doctor

———∽∾∾∽———

In your quest for diagnosis and treatment of your migraines, you need to find the best physician possible. So how do you do that?

Although there are many ways to find a physician who treats migraines, we think the place to start is with a qualified neurologist. So how do you find him or her?

Often, one has only to look in the phone book under the heading of "physicians" to find a neurologist—although we do *not* recommend randomly selecting your doctor from the phone book listings. The number of physicians available for you to choose from also varies depending on where you live. For example, in most larger cities, several neurologists practice in the given area while in less populated areas there may be no neurologists for hundreds of miles. We think that at least your initial visit or two should be with a neurologist. Then, if geography makes frequent visits impractical, the local family practitioner can be the designated treating physician.

If you already have a family practitioner or internist, then certainly this question should be put to your doctor: Who is a good neurologist? Probably your doctor will also know a good neurologist with some interest in migraine (not all neurologists are intrigued by migraines). If a referral of this nature is not possible, then obtaining the name from a friend who is seeing a neurologist and is satisfied with the care would be another good referral possibility.

Occasionally there will be a neurologist in your area who has published work on migraine that you can examine in order to determine if this physician is right for you. Also hospitals frequently have hotlines or printed material on specialists such as neurologists, but we urge caution here because hospitals often promote physicians who support the hospital's interest. Those interests may or may not coincide with yours.

A visit with a neurologist will not be inexpensive. However, the reason for the visit should be held in sharp focus. The cost of visiting the physician should be compared to lost wages and direct suffering related to the headache, as well as the suffering endured by the entire family when one member is severely affected by an illness of this nature.

Approach your physician with an open mind, but if it becomes clear during the interview or the examination that this physician is "just not right" for you, then try again. Keep in mind that migraine is a chronic illness, thus it is desirable that your relationship with your physician will last for many years.

Frequently patients will go to a neurologist chosen by the gatekeeper of their HMO, stating: "I have no other choice." While we do not choose our parents, siblings, or children, we can choose our spouses, friends, and, in our opinion equally important, our physicians.

While it might be reasonable to see the neurologist in your HMO initially, one should clearly have no compulsion to continue with that physician if a good patient-doctor climate is not achieved within one or two visits. Paying the neurologist's fee out of your own pocket when outside the HMO will often pay for itself many times over by saving you from pain thus giving you more time for work and other pursuits.

So how do we go about making the right match? What is it about one physician as compared to another that makes him or her a good physician or, more importantly, the right physician for you?

Let's explain with an illustration. We perform many free educational seminars on back pain, neck pain, and migraine disorders, which we start with the sub-theme that open communication between the patient and doctor is essential.

One popular slide we use at our seminars pictures a golfer standing in a sand trap, looking up and asking a friend for a sand wedge. His friend hands down a sandwich to the baffled golfer.

If you find yourself constantly asking your physician for a sand wedge yet you continue to receive a sandwich, there is a lack of communication between you and your doctor.

Some Simple Guidelines

To get the most from each encounter with your physician, we suggest several guidelines:

- Be prepared. Know what your problem is or what your concerns are. Write them down. Bring any x-rays, medications, information on past medical interventions, and any information you have on your headache history. How old were you when they started? How severe was the first episode? How many headaches are you having per month or week? What seems to work? What doesn't?

- Ask the doctor if he or she is comfortable treating acute and chronic migraineurs. Not everyone is. For

example, some doctors state "I don't give out narcotics" as a pat response to pain management.

- Ask the doctor about how many migraine patients
he or she treats in a year. Some doctors are not very
experienced in treating this disorder and may provide
elaborate explanations and little practical advice.

- Ask the doctor if he or she treats migraines with a
variety of medications. If the doctor is resistant to
trying new medications, this may be the wrong
physician for you.

We often compare the doctor-patient relationship to a mar-
riage, with the physician's office as the bedroom. Specifically, it
is an intimate place, where very important questions and
actions are undertaken, and frank, open, and honest discus-
sions regarding specific needs take place.

You need to be willing to share information and to be a
partner in your own health care. Be honest about what you can
and cannot do when it comes to treating your pain syndrome.

For example, one patient has assured us for four years
now that she will immediately discontinue smoking if "You
can just get me through this headache." But she has continued to use tobacco, which is a notorious trigger for headache
disorders. I've explained many times that this habit may be
playing a role in her migraine suffering, but this patient is
comfortable with a "quick fix" and is not interested in resolving the underlying problem.

On the other hand, some people just cannot remove certain triggers or life stressors. It's important to be honest with
your doctor about that as well. For example, if you have a difficult boss and a stressful work environment, and you have no
way of leaving your work station to abort an acute migraine,
tell your doctor. It does you no good if a treatment plan is
carefully outlined when you know there's no chance you can
follow it. Tell your physicians that you can't comply and ask
for another option.

Doctors Are Human!

It's also a good idea to remember that your doctor is a person, not a god. Still, the physician does not like to be challenged in a mean or nasty way, such as "Doctor, don't you know the latest information on that?" or "Doctor, I just saw 60 Minutes. I think that medicine will kill me!"

Instead, an assertive and positive statement such as, "Doctor, I understand there may be some side effects to this. Can you explain them to me?" or "Doctor, I'm concerned about some information I saw on TV last night regarding the medication you just prescribed. Can you explain why you want to use it? What are the side effects, and what can I expect?"

In a spirit of cooperation, mountains can be moved and migraines can be removed—if you work together with your doctor.

Evaluating a Prospective Physician for Yourself

What else constitutes a good match?

- Punctuality may be an indicator. If you are notoriously late and the doctor you see is notoriously on time, or vice-versa, then this may not be a good match.
- See how the staff treats you. *If* the first question out of a staff person's mouth is "How are you going to pay for this?" you may assume that money is the key issue here.

On the other hand, if the physician's staff asks for information in a pleasant way—for example, requests prior records, x-rays, documents, and so forth—you can be at least somewhat reassured that this doctor's primary concern is to get as much information as possible to come up with the correct diagnosis for you.

- Of course, your doctor's visit *will* cost you some money, and if there are particular financial needs that you have, it's a good idea to ask about the office financial policy on the first visit. Questions such as "Is there an installment policy?" or "Does the doctor bill the insurance company directly?" or "About how much can I expect the office visit to cost?" are all reasonable and appropriate to ask.

Sometimes you may have been referred to the new doctor by a friend, preferably someone with a similar problem who has done well with the physician you're planning to see. But do keep in mind that personalities are all different, and what one person likes in a doctor, another person may dislike intensely.

The bottom line is that you need to feel comfortable with the doctor and have confidence that he or she understands your problem and will listen to your complaints and try to do something about them. Do keep in mind, however, that if you've already seen twenty-five doctors, it is almost certain that there will be nothing magical about Doctor Number 26.

Health care is a precious resource and needs to be investigated thoroughly by prospective patients. You would not buy a new car (we hope!) without doing at least a little research. Nor should you trust your health to any doctor without doing a background check, office inspection, and even an initial evaluation to determine if this is going to be a positive experience.

Keep in mind that migraine pain is miserable enough without having to battle uphill with a physician.

9

Your Neurological Exam and Tests Your Doctor May Order

———— ❧❧❧ ————

It's a good idea to have some advance knowledge of what medical information and documentation your new doctor will probably want you to bring with you to your first neurological exam, what kinds of questions he or she is likely to ask, and what types of tests your physician may order.

What to Bring to the Exam

When you visit your neurologist for the first time, besides bringing with you a positive attitude, you should be sure to bring medical records from other physicians who have treated you for other problems, including problems which don't seem to relate to your headaches or migraines.

Why? Because records that you may regard as irrelevant and unimportant may actually be very valuable to the physician who will try to help you with your migraines. And if the doctor does not need the information, that's okay too. It's better to bring "too much" than too little.

Important note: Plan ahead. Be sure to give yourself enough time to obtain those records. Call your other doctor(s) at least a week ahead of time whenever possible and find out when you may pick up the information and who can give it to you (that's usually whoever is in charge of medical records or the x-ray department).

Explain to the staff that the neurologist you were referred to is asking for complete medical records.

Keep in mind that sometimes doctors' offices do not like to release information directly to patients and consequently may insist on sending your records straight to the neurologist. The problem with this is that sending out medical records to Doctor B may be a low priority to Doctor A's staff—so low that they forget to do it.

If the staff absolutely refuses to release your records to you—and appealing directly to the doctor (their boss) doesn't help, then politely ask the staff when the records will be mailed. Be sure to call the neurologist's office before your appointment to make sure they actually received your records. (As a last resort, provide your new physician's fax number—you would be surprised by how many faxed records we receive on patients the day of their visits.)

Records that you *must* bring are your x-rays and MRIs. These are very important to the neurologist. Bring actual MRI films or CAT scans instead of written radiological reports because most neurologists are skilled at reading CAT scans as well as MRIs and may find abnormalities not observed by radiologists.

Cooperate as Much as Possible

Not to overstate the case, but remember to hold onto your positive mental attitude. Keep in mind that the doctor's goal is to empower you; and as you begin the diagnostic process with the physician, the responsibility for a satisfactory outcome is shared. Your good health care must be perceived as a joint doctor-patient goal. Think of yourself as providing evidence that your doctor will interpret, Sherlock Holmes–like, as clues to your diagnosis.

The initial phase of the "investigation" will consist of the clinical history. As is common with many other chronic problems, migraine is often diagnosed, at least in part, with the use of a questionnaire. (See the appendix for an example of a commonly used headache questionnaire.)

Certainly a questionnaire does not take the place of an intelligent doctor-patient dialog. The neurologist would much rather explore the nature of your complaints and precise responses (the best you can give) to the questions than hear a self-diagnosis. In other words, telling your doctor "I'm here because I have migraine" is not particularly helpful.

Even patients who suffer from migraines do not have their diagnosis stamped indelibly on their foreheads. Physicians must consider hundreds of possible conditions that could be causing the headaches. Failure to identify a serious, treatable cause of headache because you withheld requested information could be catastrophic for you.

Questions Neurologists Ask

The physician will ask you when your symptoms started, how frequent they are, how long they last (minutes, hours, days?), and how severe they are. The doctor also needs to know about associated symptoms preceding, accompanying, or following the actual attacks. As has been mentioned elsewhere in this book, the diagnosis of migraine is based more on the recognition of a pattern of symptoms rather than on any one specific symptom or physical finding.

What medications are you now taking?   Lists of your medications as well as their effects on the migraine and their side effects will be of great interest to your physician. You might actually bring the medications in to show the doctor, so he or she can check the exact dosage, timing, and so on.

Are you affected by external factors that seem to trigger your migraines? Trigger factors are of particular interest. These may include habits such as smoking, or drinking alcohol or caffeinated beverages, as well as patterns of sleep, work, and sexual activity. (See chapter 6 on non-food migraine triggers.)

What is your emotional state? Your general emotional state, as well as the emotional state you experience during migraine attacks will be of interest to a skilled neurologist. Normal nervousness is okay, and the doctor knows that.

What is your medical history? This will be explored in great detail, to help in diagnosing as well as in deciding what medication you should be treated with.

For example, doctors will not prescribe the medication Inderal for patients with asthma. Patients with severe coronary artery disease would not be candidates for ergotamine or some of the other therapies frequently used in migraine treatment. Why not? Because these medications can lead to reduced blood flow to the heart or irregularities of the heart rate that would be dangerous for people with such illnesses.

Your physician is also likely to explore your family history (including your parents', siblings', possibly your children's) at length. Since relevant data are often not uncovered during the first visit (despite the best intentions of both patient and neurologist), the doctor will update your history at subsequent visits.

Be open with your physician, and don't be offended by questions related to tobacco, alcohol, street drugs, sexually transmitted disease, or sexual habits. The doctor needs this information to provide you with an accurate diagnosis and the best possible care.

The important thing to remember is that your medical history and your responses to the doctor's questions are the basis for making an accurate diagnosis of migraine. Although tests may confirm the findings or provide additional helpful information, we can't overestimate the value of a thorough medical history in diagnosing your condition and getting you on the path to improved health.

The Physical Exam

After completion of the history, the physician will begin the examination. We prefer to examine patients in a partially unclothed state. A gown is provided to the patient prior to the physical examination.

Initially, the neurologist will examine the cranium for evidence of local disease such as sinusitis, or tender scalp or arteries. The jaw joints are examined as are the eyes and eardrums. A brief examination of the teeth, mouth, throat, and so on is also performed. The physician is likely to examine various portions of the cranium as well as the neck and heart with a stethoscope. We also look for any abnormalities of the skin.

The Neurological Physical Exam

After a general physical examination, the physician will conduct the formal neurologic examination. This will include obtaining some idea of the patient's emotional state, intelligence, verbal skills, and thought organization. Simple tests of memory, abstraction, and more complex use of language are frequently given to supplement the mental status examination. You're not being given an "IQ" test so don't worry about giving the "wrong" answer. Just answer honestly.

Next the physician will undertake the cranial nerve examination to assess sensation in your face, movement of your face and tongue, as well as your sight and hearing. He or she will examine the retina of your eye with a device called an ophthalmoscope. Motor strength and coordination are tested as are the reflexes, the ability to perceive vibration, and other tactile stimuli. Don't be surprised if the doctor tells you to walk around the room or even in the hallway, since it's important to examine how you walk.

The Next Step for the Doctor

What happens next will depend on a number of factors. In cases in which the patient has a long, well-documented history of a benign headache condition such as migraine and has already had relevant testing including CT or MRI of the brain, no additional studies may be considered. However, in most cases of chronic headaches, the treating physician will usually order further tests. Generally, some blood tests and an MRI will be ordered, although other tests may be indicated too.

Neurological Tests

There is some controversy about the necessity of tests in patients with garden variety migraine and who present a normal neurological examination. If your neurologist decides further testing is needed, often he or she will order imaging studies such as MRI or CAT scan of the brain. Since further tests may be indicated, we'll talk about those as well.

CAT Scans

The CAT scan (sometimes referred to by doctors as the "CT" scan) is a painless special kind of x-ray. Until the arrival and general acceptance of MRI scans, the CAT scan was the "gold standard" of brain imaging. Excellent views of the cranium and its contents can be obtained with this advanced technology. Hemorrhages, strokes, tumors, and increased intercranial pressure are frequently suggested by the CAT scans. In a patient with migraine, however, the CAT scans are generally normal.

Magnetic Resonance Imaging (MRI)

The MRI has proved to be a virtual revolution in medical diagnosis, particularly in relation to diagnosis of disorders of the brain and spine. When an imaging study is indicated in a patient with migraine, we favor this study because of its superior resolution and greater flexibility over CAT scans.

Please note: If you have had an MRI in the past, that doesn't necessarily mean you don't need another one. For example, your previous MRI may have been done years ago, or it may have been for a part of the body other than the head.

This type of technology is excellent for demonstrating stroke, most hemorrhages, and tumors, and frequently MRIs can actually reveal areas with subtle reduced blood flow—a common finding in the MRIs of patients with migraine. Abnormal blood vessels, which are frequently not seen on a CAT scan, often show up with excellent resolution on an MRI.

Intravenous dye material (don't worry, it's safe!), which provides better image contrast between abnormalities and normal brain tissue, is frequently given intravenously prior to completion of the study. More often than not, MRIs in patients with uncomplicated migraine are entirely normal.

What is an MRI like? The patient is enclosed in a chamber-like machine for this painless test. For the majority of patients, it's no big deal. However, some individuals experience claustrophobia-like symptoms—often people who never knew they were claustrophobic—and need to be medicated ahead of time with Valium or some other calming sedative. In some cases, patients are disturbed by the droning noise of the machine.

In our experience, about 15–20 percent of patients need some type of sedation when undergoing the MRI test. There does seem to be a technological trend toward less-enclosed MRI scanners; however, at present, we do not believe they are widely available. Our experience to date has been that the quality of the scan is not as good with these newer devices; however, advances in technology should rectify this problem.

With all its many advantages, however, the MRI will tell us little about inflammation in blood vessels and infectious processes, both of which frequently have headache as a prominent symptom.

The MRI is the most costly of the tests described in this chapter and can run about $1,200 or more.

Electrically Based Tests

Prior to the advent of advanced diagnostic imaging studies such as CAT scans and MRI, electrophysiologic (electric) tests were routinely used on patients with headaches. While this type of examination frequently turns up some useful data, it is still a crude technology when directed to the task of investigating structural lesions of the brain.

The electroencephalogram (EEG), the most commonly used electrophysiologic study of the brain, can be abnormal during a migraine attack. In this test, electrodes are placed on the scalp and brain wave patterns are measured by a machine. This is a painless test, and often patients fall asleep during the testing process. There is also a 24-hour EEG test, in which the patient carries around a portable machine, but such a test is almost never used by neurologists to evaluate headaches.

Usually the EEG between migraine attacks is normal; however, there may be some subtle changes. For example, certain features of migraine can be quite bizarre and are often suggestive of some type of epileptic phenomenon. The EEG is quite helpful in this regard. Abnormal EEGs are extremely common during an actual migraine attack.

Visual Evoked Potentials

This test has been available for about thirty years, although many lay people have probably never heard of it. It is not used frequently but may be indicated if a patient reports visual changes or has an atypical history.

Visual evoked potentials is a complex electrophysiologic test that allows the physician to test how fast and how well an image is transmitted from the eye to the portion of the brain involved with seeing (the occipital region). Sometimes injury to the optic pathways can cause visual complaints, and this test allows the physician to measure several different potentials.

During this test, the patient looks at a checkerboard that changes in some way, such as from black to white. Electrodes on the head will record the "potential" or impulse at various sites.

Certain abnormalities in this test are seen on a fairly frequent basis in patients with migraine. However, it must be emphasized that a normal or abnormal visual evoked potential does not with certainty confirm or rule out the diagnosis of migraine.

Angiography

Angiography is a test that allows indirect examination of blood vessels. This can be used for the head, neck, or other portions of the body. As a general rule, this test is not recommended for patients with a normal CAT scan or MRI. However, it can be important if there is some suggestion by history, physical examination, or (on the MRI) of some type of abnormal blood vessel, usually an AVM (arterial venous malformation), which is an abnormal connection between the arterial and venous blood supplies.

The angiogram involves some type of arterial puncture, usually in the groin area. A tiny tube is inserted up through the artery that leads into the aorta of the heart and then into the blood vessels of the brain. Dye is inserted through the tube to provide better contrast to show up in x-rays. Then x-rays in multiple planes are obtained, giving a three-dimensional indication of the size, location, and often the nature of the vessel in question. This test can be somewhat painful, although many patients report that it's not much worse than a blood test. The average test can take up to an hour.

Frequently the walls of abnormal blood vessels are thin and easily ruptured, which can lead to headache or even a stroke or severe neurologic dysfunction and possibly death. That is why advance diagnosis of such a condition is so important. The angiogram can provide this crucial information.

More recently, MRA (magnetic resonance angiography) has become available. It is not clear at this point if this type of procedure will replace conventional angiography described previously.

There has been some suggestion in the literature in the past that angiography in migraineurs carries an increased risk of injury to the brain. This risk has been borne out by definitive studies.

Thermography

Many physicians consider a thermography examination to be primarily punitive. Usually the patient is asked to disrobe and put on a skimpy garment much like a thong bikini. The patient is placed before a heat-sensitive camera during three sessions in which the emission of heat from various portions of the body is measured. About 60 percent of all migraineurs have a "cold patch" on their bodies between attacks. A cold patch is a small, well-demarcated area of reduced heat emission.

While results of this study are frequently abnormal during a migraine attack, the absolute diagnostic significance of the test is still far from clear. As a result, we rarely order this test. We note it here as a possible test that your physician may order.

Lumbar Puncture

Lumbar puncture (spinal tap) is rarely a reasonable measure in the diagnosis of migraine. In the spinal tap, the fluid (cerebrospinal fluid) that surrounds the brain and spinal cord is withdrawn with a needle placed in the lower back area. This test can be mildly painful, although a competent physician should be able to perform the test with minimal pain to the patient.

Chemical and microscopic examination of the fluid is often quite helpful for a diagnosis of diseases related to the brain. For example, many types of infection present very characteristic abnormalities in the composition of the cerebrospinal fluid. The content and composition of this fluid is normal between and usually even during migraine attacks. However, it is not unusual for abnormal cells to be found in the cerebrospinal fluid of patients suffering from an acute migraine attack. This test usually serves to exclude certain conditions from consideration such as hemorrhage, infection, or other inflammatory condition affecting the brain.

Laboratory Testing

If your doctor suspects there may be an inflammation of blood vessels of the brain, laboratory tests for arteritis or vasculitis, both inflammations of the blood vessels, can be ordered.

Conclusion

The most critical aspect of the diagnostic assessment is the patient history, and the most critical component of that history is the patient. Be as honest and accurate as you can. If you don't know an answer, it is all right to say so; but if you can, find the answer and report back later. Remember, this is not an inquisition, this is hopefully an establishment of a good ongoing relationship between you and your doctor—with the mutual goal of improving your health.

10

Medications for Migraine

"The desire to take medication is perhaps the greatest feature that separates man from animals."—*Sir William Osler*

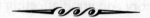

The Not-So-Good Old Days

When people in ancient civilizations suffered from migraines, the "cure" might have been trepanning (drilling holes in the skull, often without any anesthesia), bloodletting after a careful placement of blood-sucking leeches, and/or dosing the patient with a wide variety of herbs, roots, and berries—generally foul-tasting concoctions. (Some people apparently believed the worse the medicine tasted, the more effective it must be.) Ancient Babylonian priests created a mixture of burnt human bones mixed with cedar oil to rub on the migraineur.

One treatment used in the first century A.D. involved the physician placing a hot iron against the forehead, which at the least probably distracted the person from the headache pain. Some people thought pressing and rubbing the throbbing area with garlic was effective.

There have also been a wide variety of cure-alls for bodily ailments ranging from headaches to stomachaches to you-name-it. In the fourteenth and fifteenth centuries, for example, powdered Egyptian mummy dust was considered a very effective medicinal all-purpose treatment for what ailed you and was particularly favored by European monarchs. (It didn't work. In fact, it made people vomit.)

Various drugs such as marijuana, cocaine, and others that are now considered dangerous and illegal have been used throughout the ages for people suffering from virtually any illness. Alcoholic substances have been popular through the generations, as have been concoctions containing alcohol. Victorian women with "sick headaches" would have been shocked if they knew they were imbibing alcohol. Or maybe they wouldn't have cared. Migraine is definitely a leveler.

This chapter covers the lawful and effective medications we rely upon today to treat people experiencing acute attacks as well as recurrent migraines.

This chapter will give you an overview of the broad array of over-the-counter (OTC) and prescribed medications—what works, their primary side effects, and important aspects to keep in mind about each medication. Also, remember that if one medication does not work, another or sometimes a combination of medications may be what you need.

In addition, the timing of medication can be important. Often if you wait too long—until you feel like your head is splitting open—it's too late for many medications to work. There is a significant time lag between the medication getting into your system and being able to attack the problem.

The route of the medication is another major determinant in how well and how fast it works. Oral medication may take an hour or longer to have an effect and is frequently complicated (as previously discussed) by a slowing down of the stomach's function during migraine attacks. Intravenous injection (direct injection into a vein), subcutaneous injection (immediately under the skin), and nasal administration (inhaling) typically result in far more efficient delivery of the medication and have effect within minutes.

Think of medications as soldiers fighting on your behalf. Send your "troops" into battle to assist you before you're too weak and debilitated to truly benefit! It is far better strategy to act when you feel a headache coming on by trying to prevent it or at least alleviate some of the pain. Of course, if for some reason you are unable to take a medication when you feel a migraine coming on, it is worthwhile to take something whenever you can. In addition, some medications, particularly those that are injectable, are very fast-acting.

Another reason you want to treat the migraine as soon as possible is that a trip to the emergency room of your local hospital can often be a nightmarish affair, not to mention a humiliating experience. Why? Because ER doctors and nurses are running around trying to help people with strokes, heart attacks, gunshot wounds, and other major trauma. They may be insensitive to the exquisite agony of the migraine headache, thinking, hey, it's "just" a headache.

In addition, a common tactic of drug abusers is to show up in a hospital emergency room complaining of headache and insisting on a shot of Demerol or some other narcotic. If you are viewed with somewhat jaundiced eyes in the emergency room, this is probably because the staff is attempting to evaluate whether or not you are on the level.

Over-the-Counter Pain Relievers

We've all heard of the most common pain relievers for migraine and other bodily ailments—acetaminophen (Tylenol), aspirin (Bayer, Excedrin), ibuprofen (Advil, Motrin) and most recently, naproxen sodium (Naprosyn, Aleve).

These medications can help if they are taken early on in an attack and in sufficient dosage to be successful. Which of these your doctor recommends depends on your medical history. For example, if you have a history of bleeding ulcers, your doctor will probably recommend you take Tylenol and avoid the other over-the-counter medications discussed here. Why? Because the others can contribute to gastritis (irritation and inflammation of the stomach lining) and stomach ailments.

How much is enough? If you choose to take aspirin, an initial dose of 650 to 975 mg should be taken as soon as possible. Tylenol users should take 1000 mg, which is the equivalent of two "Extra-Strength" tablets.

Keep in mind that because these medications are taken orally, the medication does not go directly from the mouth into the bloodstream and attack your pain problem. Instead, it must pass through the esophagus (food tube) and stomach to the small intestine, the site of absorption, and finally to the area needing pain relief.

Peak blood levels (which indicate when the medication is working at its best level) of aspirin in non-migrainous individuals is about two hours. But if the person is suffering from migraine, the medication's action is slowed down considerably.

Another problem is that you may be vomiting so much that you lose all or most of the medication you've taken. However, you can combat this problem by supplementing your aspirin, acetaminophen, or other over-the-counter medication with an anti-nausea prescription medication known as metoclopramide (Reglan). Not only will this medication keep you from vomiting, but it will also speed the transmission of the painkillers through your system. Reglan is most effective when given through intramuscular or intravenous injections.

There are other medicines, of course, that physicians use rather than Reglan, but many studies have revealed that Reglan is quite effective in migraine headache management. One special protocol uses Reglan with an additional prescription medication to abort migraine symptoms.

This treatment may have to be repeated a few times for maximum effectiveness because the Reglan may wear off before the migraine chemical change has completely resolved. However, just knowing that there are medicines out there that can actually reduce the nausea and vomiting as well as relieve the overall suffering is sometimes enough to enable the migraine sufferer to endure an acute attack. Certainly, knowing such treatment is available should reduce the anxiety many migraine sufferers experience with the onset of symptoms.

Commonly Used Medications—News Flash!

The latest information as of summer 1995 reveals that even deficiencies of trace minerals such as magnesium can produce severe intractable headache pain. As a result, an adequate replacement of magnesium often leads to complete cessation of the severe migraine attack. That a natural substance can offer a cure is exciting news.

For migraine headache sufferers who have only trace deficiencies of magnesium, oftentimes oral replacement of the magnesium or multivitamin therapy with low-dose magnesium can be helpful in alleviating the patient's headache pain.

As noted in *Neurology 45* (supplement 4, April 1995), magnesium sulfate given intravenously to patients with a low serum magnesium level significantly reduced their severe headache pain.

Sumatriptan: The Miracle Medication

Sumatriptan (Imitrex), available in oral and subcutaneous preparations, represents nothing short of a revolution in the treatment of acute migraine. The subcutaneous administration can stop a headache cold in a dramatic manner since it gets into the system much faster than the oral preparation, and patients can be taught to self-administer sumatriptan by injecting it directly under their skin.

One problem is that often the headache recurs within 24 hours. Side effects of this medication are usually benign:

lightheadedness, flushing, weakness, and, occasionally, nausea and vomiting. Sometimes mild blood-pressure increases occur. Patients over age 45 should receive an electrocardiogram (EKG) before having this medication prescribed.

While sumatriptan (Imitrex) has been formulated in oral and subcutaneous preparations, only the subcutaneous preparations may be prescribed in the United States as of this writing.

This medication has been touted even more than aspirin as the wonder drug of today. It can often alleviate not only the migraine headache in twelve to twenty minutes, but also the uncomfortable side effects, such as the malaise or fatigue as well as the nausea and cramping of the stomach that often occur with migraine.

The pharmaceutical company that manufactures Imitrex has created an auto-injector that patients can carry discreetly, for example in a purse. As a result, if patients are squeamish about giving themselves an actual injection, the auto-injector can do that for them without their ever having to view a needle. If the auto-injector is not required, often a half-dose (3 mg) has been effective in our experience, and this dosage can be repeated.

We caution patients to be forthright, however, regarding their medical history—especially any history of chest pain or any suspicion of coronary artery disease—before we allow use of this medication. Why? Because there are reports of narrowing of the heart arteries with the use of the Imitrex injection. Despite this potential problem, we have found that Imitrex is an extremely effective medication that we have used safely in our office as well as in the hospital emergency room.

One patient, a young woman who works as an administrative assistant, was quite pleased with the initiation of Imitrex, which essentially changed her life. She had been averaging three to four migraines per month and required two to four days of disability time off each month. She was becoming very frustrated, as was her employer.

Now, she carries the Imitrex injections in her purse, and when she feels a headache "coming on," she leaves her office, goes to the ladies room, and in the privacy of a stall, gives herself an injection. She stays there for about ten minutes and then returns to her desk. No one knows that she ever had a sick headache.

She recently informed us that she has had a promotion! Because she has had no more absences from work, the quality of her work has increased, and she's become a more comprehensive "team player." She has been rewarded. Her life is considerably happier.

Nonsteroidal Anti-Inflammatory Medications (NSAIDS)

The prototype of this important group of medications was aspirin, and the lower doses of over-the-counter medications such as Motrin, Aleve, and others have already been mentioned.

Migraineurs may need larger doses (for example, as much as a 750 to 1000 mg dose of Naprosyn), which are available by prescription only. Medications frequently used in higher doses by physicians include ibuprofen (Motrin), diclofenac sodium (Voltaren), naproxen sodium (Naprosyn), ketorolac (Toradol), as well as many others.

We have had great success with Daypro, an anti-inflammatory medicine that can be given as a once-a-day dosing regimen. It is important to understand that there are many classes of anti-inflammatory medicines, all acting on a slightly different chemical basis. It is also important to understand which anti-inflammatory medication your doctor prescribes, as there are many medicines in each class.

For example, if a medication from one class didn't work for you, it might be better to switch to a different class of anti-inflammatory medications altogether rather than to try using other medicines in the first class.

Medication use is often confusing for patients and is even confusing for physicians at times. That is why it is crucial for patients to keep as accurate a diary as possible of medicines that have worked or failed in the past. Then a new physician doesn't have to start from "square one."

A new and exciting addition to this class of medications is Toradol, which is available both orally and as an intramuscular injection. Often injected doses of 60 mg of Toradol can ward off a severe migrainous attack.

Caffeine is also used in treating migraine headaches, either alone or in conjunction with other medications. We don't really know how caffeine works, but it does appear to have its own pain-relieving effect in migraine. Possibly, this effect is related to increased alertness and improved mood, or it may also be related to the dilation of cranial blood vessels. However, keep in mind that if you abruptly discontinue caffeine consumption (for example, the heavy coffee drinker decides to give up coffee completely), this could actually cause severe headaches. Why? Because your body is used to it, and you're depriving your body of what it expects.

Some medications are combined with caffeine and also butalbital, which is a barbiturate related to phenobarbital. The butalbital probably works to alleviate anxiety.

Butalbital may also be very effective as a muscle relaxer, relaxing the muscles over the base of the skull surrounding the cranium and also at the back side of the neck. Almost invariably, when patients suffer from severe migraine, their neck muscles tighten up and they feel stiff and sore. The butalbital almost always improves this problem. We have had a great deal of success with the medication Esgic Plus.

But unfortunately, butalbital as well as some other types of barbiturates have the tendency to create a habit-forming dependency, which is always a concern when a person has frequent headaches and needs to use a medication on a routine basis.

Medications that contain barbiturates are not recommended for people who suffer from major depression. Also keep in mind that butalbital can definitely impair your ability to drive or operate heavy equipment, as it may cause significant sedation.

Midrin

Midrin is a compound medication that includes acetaminophen and dichloralphenazone, a gentle sedative. These medications are combined with isometheptene mucate, which helps constrict the blood vessels and reduce head pain.

We have used Midrin successfully for several years and have seen numerous patients with fairly severe migraine greatly helped by this medication. Keep in mind, however, that "rebound headaches" can occur if this medication is used more than two or three times per week. A rebound headache is a headache caused by overuse of the medication itself.

It's also important to know that isometheptene mucate can be dangerous for patients who suffer from high blood pressure, liver or kidney disease, or glaucoma.

Anti-Emetics (Anti-Nausea Medications)

Anti-emetics are frequently invaluable in treating the acute attack because they enable the patient to keep the medication down so it can do its job. Also, since nausea and vomiting are sometimes the worst part of the illness for the patient, avoiding this aspect is quite a relief.

Anti-emetics include such medications as Reglan, Thorazine, Phenergan, Compazine, Tigan, and others that are available in oral and injectable forms, as well as in suppository form.

Side effects of the anti-emetics do occur, and the key ones are abnormal involuntary movements, reduced blood pressure, drowsiness, and anxiety. Sometimes more serious problems occur, such as liver disease, allergies, dermatitis (skin rashes), gastroenteritis, and even bone marrow suppression. Fortunately, the severe side effects are quite rare.

Ergotamine

A mainstay of the acute migraine attack, ergotamine has proven effective for about half of all patients suffering from migraines. This medication can be administered rectally, orally, or by placing a tablet under the tongue (sublingually).

Oral medications include Cafergot and Wigraine, which contain 1 mg of ergotamine and 100 mg of caffeine. Typically, two tablets are taken as early as possible during the headache and may be repeated every thirty minutes to a maximum of six tablets per day.

When discussing ergotamine or ergot medications, one must remember that too much of a good medication is not a good thing. We always want to carefully monitor the risks vs. the benefits of any medication. And, as previously noted, individuals with other medical conditions can have problems taking this type of medication.

The ergots have a tendency to cause blood vessel contractions. We have found that in our patients, both the veins and arteries are affected when doses high enough to produce any benefit or pain relief are used. As a result, if ergotamines are used, it is very important to be sure that your blood pressure is monitored, and also to ensure that a steadily increasing dosage of the ergotamine is not needed to control your symptoms.

The Bellergal-S preparation contains 0.3 mg of ergotamine, 0.2 mg of belladonna, and 40 mg of phenobarbitol. One tablet is administered orally at the onset of the headache and may be repeated again after an eight-hour period. Since these pills are strong, no more than two can be taken each day.

The rectal preparations of ergotamine are Cafergot suppositories and Wigraine suppositories, and they contain 2 mg of ergotamine and 100 mg of caffeine. One or one-and-a-half suppositories (depending on your doctor's direction) is inserted rectally at the onset of the headache and may be repeated after one hour. No more than two of these suppositories can be taken in a day. One trick that we have found is to try one quarter or one half of a suppository at the headach onset rather than one full suppository. This can then be repeated every 4 to 6 hours for symptom relief.

Sublingual preparations of ergotamine include Ergomar and Ergostat, each of which contains 2 mg of ergotamine. The medication is placed under the tongue at the beginning of a headache and may be repeated every half hour up to three tablets per day.

The main side effect of the ergotamines are nausea and vomiting, which can be relieved by prior administration of Reglan. Less frequent side effects are dizziness, muscle cramping, tingling, diarrhea, and abdominal cramps. Occasional side effects are drowsiness, chest pain, shortness of breath, fainting, and limb pain.

Patients with severe atherosclerosis, coronary artery disease, and high blood pressure should stay away from this medication. In addition, if you have hyperthyroid disease, are pregnant, or are a nursing mother, avoid this medication.

Despite the wide spectrum of side effects that can come with ergotamine, this medication is often considered a godsend to patients who suffer from frequent and debilitating migraine attacks.

Dihydroergotamine (DHE)

Dihydroergotamine is a safe and effective medication, which until recently was the unchallenged "gold standard" for the treatment of an established migraine attack. While chemically similar to ergotamine, it appears to be less constrictive of the blood vessels. In addition, unlike ergotamine, DHE is often very effective when the patient is in the throes of a severe attack.

DHE is administered intravenously or intramuscularly, and a nasally administered preparation is on the horizon for those patients who are squeamish about injections. Injection usually follows 10 mg of intravenous Reglan. Often patients can be taught to self-administer DHE, thus avoiding the hospital emergency room.

Nausea is a common problem with DHE, and patients may sometimes also suffer the side effects of sedation, anxiety, diarrhea, and body aches. DHE is not recommended for patients with significant coronary disease or poorly controlled hypertension. Nor is DHE recommended for pregnant women.

Note: Any woman who thinks she may be pregnant should absolutely consult her physician prior to taking any anti-migraine medications, including over-the-counter medicines as simple as aspirin or Motrin. Although generally safe and effective, these medications can have side effects that may be significant in women who are pregnant.

Narcotics

Many physicians are hesitant to prescribe narcotics for migraines, although most neurologists use this type of medication at some point in their careers. The problem is that studies have revealed the risk of addiction in patients with migraine is high, and doctors do not want to add the problem of addiction to the existing problem of recurrent migraines.

Narcotics prescribed by physicians for migraines usually include various compound formulations of aspirin or acetaminophen combined with propoxyphene, oxycodone, or some other synthetic chemical. Examples of the proprietary medications of this type are Darvocet, Darvon, Percodan, Percocet, Vicodin, and Lorcet.

Since these can provide rapid relief for patients who are in severe pain or who are truly unable to tolerate other medications, they may provide a temporary solution for the migraineur.

An additional commonly used narcotic is Tylenol with Codeine, with varying dosages of codeine.

Stadol

Besides the oral medications already described, a new nasal spray has been introduced (Stadol NS). This medication is convenient, safe, and frequently effective for an acute attack of migraine.

Patients should be aware that continued, frequent use of these medications poses risk. For this reason physicians are loath to use them indiscriminately. Nonetheless, this is often a temporary solution for rapid relief in patients experiencing severe pain who are unable to tolerate other medications or for whom other medications have been unsuccessful.

Stadol NS has proven effective in migraine, usually acting within fifteen minutes. Approximately 43 percent of patients taking this medication complain of some somnolence (sleepiness). The convenience of this method of administration makes this a valuable tool in the treatment of an acute attack of migraine.

Unfortunately, an additional side effect of the Stadol nasal spray is some disorientation and lightheadedness if it is used incorrectly.

One common complaint from our patients is that they do not always know if they are really getting that first spray and ultimately overdose themselves by taking a second inhalation in the other nostril, thinking that the first one "didn't get through."

We find that these patients get excellent relief from their migraine pain, but they can be relatively incapacitated if they are not cautious in how they use the medication. Often education—reminders of how to use the medication effectively and simple instructions to "prime the pump"—will alleviate this problem.

Preventive Medications

If their patient suffers from recurring migraines, physicians will often decide to prescribe a preventive medication. This decision is based on the severity and frequency of the headache, as well as on factors related to the patient's medical history and his or her ability to tolerate various medications.

Many doctors recommend prophylactic (preventive) therapy for patients suffering from more than one attack a month, while others suggest treatment for those with weekly attacks.

In addition to the other-listed medicines, we feel strongly that one of the most potent therapies to an acute migraine attack is to go to sleep. This will come as no surprise to many migraine sufferers, who know that if they can just lie down in a dark quiet room and get to sleep, then often they feel much better when they awaken.

One of the medications we like to use as a sleep inducer is Ambien, which is a non-addicting, non-habit-forming sleep medication that is quite potent. There are many other sedative medications, but, unfortunately, many of them also have side effects, such as a "hung over" feeling when used on a chronic basis. We have not seen these problems with Ambien.

Another guideline for determining therapy to prevent migraine headaches is the degree and severity of disability that occurs with these headaches. If your migraine headaches don't cost you much in terms of time or money, and are tolerated by those around you, then your physician may allow a greater number per month before starting preventive therapy.

However, if even one sick headache per month produces significant disability, financial loss, or social complications, it may well indicate that it is time to try preventive treatment. Since there are no clear-cut guidelines, you should consult with your physician.

Beta Blockers

A class of medications that inhibit the effect of adrenaline and other similar compounds, beta blockers are medications that affect the heart, blood vessels, lungs, and central nervous system. The most commonly prescribed beta blocker is propranolol (Inderal). Used properly, this medication can decrease the severity, duration, and frequency of the migraine attack.

Inderal is available in a standard and also a long-acting preparation (Inderal-LA). The LA preparation can be taken once a day, but twice daily doses are usually recommended for the higher doses. We favor initiation of Inderal-LA, 80 mg per day, increasing weekly to an effective dose unless or until the medication causes unpleasant side effects. Some neurologists prescribe up to 400 mg of this medication per day, administered in divided doses.

Since Inderal is also often used to treat patients with high blood pressure, as one might expect, a side effect of this medication can be lightheadedness and low blood pressure. Inderal can also slow the heart rate and even constrict the airways. Consequently, it is dangerous for patients with emphysema or underlying asthma.

If Inderal will work for you, you'll usually notice a benefit within four weeks. Don't give up, however, until you've tried it for at least three months in as high a dose as your physician believes your system can tolerate.

You may need to take this medication for several years. Don't stop taking it suddenly, however, because an abrupt termination could lead to dangerous elevations of your blood pressure and heart rate.

Generally, any lightheadedness that you may experience decreases over several weeks, as does the diarrhea and the coldness of hands and feet that sometimes occurs with this medication.

Some people should *not* take beta blockers. Patients with severe coronary artery disease, most of those who have irregularities in their heart rate, and patients with chronic lung problems should avoid beta blockers. If you have severe narrowing of the arteries in the legs, don't take this medication, especially if you are also taking ergotamine or methysergide. Also, because of the potential slowing of pulse, we teach our patients to take their pulse. If it drops below 55 beats per minute, we often will lower the medication dose.

Diabetics should either avoid altogether or be extremely careful with beta blockers because often diabetics rely on the symptoms of sweating, anxiety, and increased heart rate to alert them to a problem with low blood sugar. Since these responses are greatly reduced in the patient on a beta blocker, this leaves the diabetic patient little margin for error in halting a severe insulin reaction.

Calcium Channel Blockers

Newer on the scene than the beta blockers are the calcium channel blockers, which are very effective medications. As with beta blockers, the key benefit of this type of medication seems to be the decrease in the frequency of the headaches, and the primary action appears to be on the blood vessels. As with Inderal, you may experience lightheadedness, flushing, and even fainting as side effects of this medication. Verapamil (Calan, Isoptin) is probably the most commonly used calcium channel blocker. Most neurologists prescribe 300 mg per day while some increase up to 480 mg per day. Higher dosages may cause swelling of the hands and feet and hand tremor. Other calcium channel blockers are nifedipine (Procardia, Adalt), nimodipine (Nimotop), diltiazem (Cardizem), and selenium (Flunarazin L), which is available in Europe but not in the United States). This category of medication can affect the efficiency of the heart's pumping and should be avoided if you have a problem with cardiac function.

Don't be surprised if you develop some ankle and leg swelling while taking moderate to high dosages of calcium channel blockers. This is an annoying side effect, and one which can often be alleviated with support stockings. In our practice, we encourage our patients to be partners in their health care, and together we determine whether or not the mild ankle swelling is more uncomfortable or annoying than are the severe migraines. We let our patients decide for themselves, with our guidance, whether or not they want to switch from the calcium channel blocker to some other form of preventive therapy.

NSAIDS

As previously discussed, NSAIDS can be used in an acute attack. They may also be given in a maintenance dose as a preventive measure. The most frequently used NSAID for this purpose is naproxen (Naprosyn) although low doses of aspirin are often used as well. The problem with taking aspirin on a daily basis (in addition to possible gastrointestinal problems) is that sometimes daily doses of aspirin lead to tension headaches. As we have already mentioned, once-a-day dosing with a medication such as Daypro often increases patient compliance and decreases stomach side effects.

Methysergide (Sansert) is another NSAID medication and one which is greatly underused as a preventive medication. One possible reason for this is that in rare cases, Sansert causes a very serious side effect, retroperitoneal fibrosis, which is formation of scar tissue in the back of the abdomen that leads to serious kidney problems. However, this rare complication can apparently be avoided by periodic drug "holidays."

An additional severe problem that Sansert may cause is some scarring of lung tissues, which can result in difficulty with breathing. This is a serious medication and should only be used under careful guidelines with the physician monitoring the patient closely.

As a result, doctors usually don't prescribe Sansert for longer than six months at a time, and they generally disrupt therapy for four to eight weeks before restarting the medication.

We use this medication if Inderal or another commonly used medication is unsuccessful. Over half the patients for whom we have prescribed Sansert respond well. The medication is usually effective within a few days.

Side effects of this medication are nausea, abdominal cramping, and diarrhea, although the side effects are usually minimized if the dosage is slowly built up over time, giving the body a chance to adjust to it. Other side effects include drowsiness, fatigue, lightheadedness, difficulty with concentration, and depression.

Patients who suffer from severe narrowing of the blood vessels in the arms and legs, or who have coronary disease or poorly controlled high blood pressure should avoid Sansert. In addition, a history of phlebitis is a good reason to steer clear of this medication.

Note: Sansert has recently been reported to be effective in migraine headaches specifically associated with menstruation. Supporters believe that starting Sansert from one to five days before the menstrual cycle and continuing the therapy until two to four days after the cycle is most effective.

Antidepressants

Even if you do not suffer from clinical depression, you may benefit from taking one of the antidepressant medications described here. The reason for this is that these medications act on and cause changes in the brain that could alleviate the pain.

Prozac is in the class of serotonin-associated medications, and is actually a serotonin uptake inhibitor. (As stated elsewhere, serotonin is a chemical messenger compound thought to play a role in migraine.)

Prozac (fluoxetine) and other medications in this class are very potent and important therapeutic interventions. However, the negative press surrounding Prozac has made many physicians reluctant to prescribe this medication for migraine rather than for major depression alone.

Many migraine sufferers experience clinical depression. This well-recognized association is addressed in several competing theories: Living with a chronic illness of any type has been shown to be a potent risk factor for depression. Moreover, some theories suggest, the migraine and the chronic daily headaches may deplete the pain-mediating neurotransmitter serotonin in significant neural populations (or possibly in some brain cells). This serotonin depletion may be a fundamental contributor to the development of depression. For these reasons, the anti-depressant Prozac holds great promise for people suffering from migraine and depression as its serotonin-repleting properties are, at least in theory, beneficial in both conditions.

Denise S. was a 25-year-old neurology resident who was greatly troubled by migraines and had only mixed results with various treatments. Adding 20 mg of Prozac twice daily improved her headaches so much that she had only one or two fairly mild attacks per year.

Initially, 20 mg of Prozac is used although doses as high as 80 mg are sometimes needed. This medication is different from most other antidepressants in that there is little if any drowsiness; instead, an increase in energy is characteristic. Weight loss may occur. We recommend this medicine not be taken close to bedtime as its stimulant effect may lead to insomnia.

We believe that Prozac is one of the most important advances in the pharmacological treatment of both depression and migraine in recent decades. The claims of the medication causing individuals to commit suicide are vastly overstated.

Traditional Antidepressants

Antidepressant medications have been around for years, and most of the older medications fall under the group of "tricyclic" or "heterocyclic," which are terms related to the chemical structure of these medications.

They have been used successfully for many years as a preventive treatment for migraineurs and their effectiveness is clearly documented in the literature, especially for amitriptyline (Elavil, Endep) and doxepin (Sinequan, Adapin). What they appear to do is influence all the major aspects of migraine headaches, including frequency, duration, and severity. Antidepressants may also be used in conjunction with other medications. For example, the combination of propranolol and amitriptyline appears to be particularly helpful.

Unfortunately, there are many side effects associated with traditional antidepressants, such as dry mouth, lightheadedness, low blood pressure, drowsiness, and difficulty with urination, particularly for older men (or men of any age with prostate enlargement).

Some traditional antidepressants, such as desipramine (Norpramin, Pertofrane), nortriptyline (Pamelor), and protriptyline (Vivactil) appear to cause less drowsiness while trazodone (Desyrel) is less likely to cause dryness of the mouth or lightheadedness.

Often these medications are prescribed to be taken at bedtime, which renders the side effects tolerable in most cases. These medications are particularly helpful when the migraine problem is complicated by actual depression.

Generally, these medications are started at a low dose which is built up gradually over several weeks. At higher doses, many of these medications can be monitored by blood levels. If they work, the effect on migraines is seen within a few weeks, although the maximum effects may not be noted for two to three months.

It's recommended that an EKG be done on patients over age 50 or those with a significant cardiac disease before starting on this medication.

Weight gain of three to five pounds or more is common with these medications. Sexual drive may be affected by traditional antidepressants, particularly in the male. Cases of priapism (a continuous and painful erection) as well as impotence have been reported.

Again, as with the serotonin agents, education plays a key role in alleviating a patient's fears when he or she begins taking a traditional antidepressant. The problem is that there is still significant stigma associated with depression and medications for depression, and physicians and patients need to overcome this obstacle.

Most of our patients are eager to try virtually any medication to prevent or alleviate their migraine disorders. When given along with education, reassurance, and instructions regarding their proper use, antidepressants can often be well tolerated and very effective for the patient.

Monoamine Oxidase Inhibitors (MAO Inhibitors)

Although we rarely use this classification of medications, it's important to provide a complete list of possible treatments.

This medication should only be used if you are a person who will unconditionally follow your physician's instructions and will report any side effects promptly.

Nardil is one common MAO inhibitor, and it may be used alone or in combination with other traditional antidepressant medications such as Elavil.

The side effects of MAO inhibitors are dramatic, when they occur. Side effects in the brain alone include occasional serious alterations in behavior, abnormal involuntary movements such as tremor and muscle twitching, and even convulsions. Fatigue is very common, as is weight gain and dryness of the mouth. Sometimes patients, particularly older men, find this medication makes it difficult to urinate. Sexual dysfunction among both men and women is a common side effect of this medication.

MAO inhibitors can also lower or increase blood pressure. An elevated blood sugar, which may result from this medication, can be difficult to control and could lead to swelling and hemorrhage of the brain, particularly in the presence of chemicals found in various foods and medications. For this reason, many foods must be avoided, including various meats and fish, avocados, bananas, tea, coffee, and chocolate.

In addition, many medications must be avoided altogether when you take an MAO inhibitor. Medications given for weight loss, asthma, or colds could lead to serious side effects when combined with an MAO inhibitor. Illegal drug use, particularly of cocaine, represents a clear danger. Narcotic pain relievers such as Demerol and even the cough suppressant dextromethorphan (present in many OCT cold medications) could lead to a severe reaction which might end in death.

If and when these medications are used, they should be avoided in patients with poorly controlled blood pressure or significant disease of the heart or brain circulation.

Cyproheptadine (Periactin)

Cyproheptadine (Periactin) is occasionally helpful in migraine prevention and is frequently cited as an effective medication for prevention of migraine in children. (See chapter 5 for more information on children and adolescents who suffer from migraines.)

This medication frequently causes drowsiness, dryness of the mouth, abdominal cramps, and urinary retention. Weight gain and increased growth in children have occasionally been seen.

An interesting case involved a 9-year-old child who was started on Periactin for his migraine headache disorder. There was strong family history of migraine, with the patient's mother having difficulty controlling her own disorder.

The child did well over a four- to six-week period of time, but gained about ten pounds and outgrew all his clothes. The mother thought that maybe the child was going through a growth spurt, but said it was peculiar for him to gain so much weight in such a short period of time.

I discussed the side effects with the mother and child, and the child volunteered that he had a constant hunger. We switched the child to a different medication, and his headache disorder remained under good control. He dropped the ten pounds—and did not need an entire new wardrobe.

Lithium

Although not a front-line medication to prevent migraine, lithium clearly does have anti-migrainous properties. Unfortunately, it is occasionally a cause of headache in its own right.

Lithium should not be prescribed by physicians inexperienced with this medication. The dosing is a complex process and the penalty (to the patient) for not doing it right can be quite severe.

Many side effects may occur with lithium. Therefore, frequent blood monitoring is required in those being treated with lithium. If the therapeutic blood levels are exceeded in lithium treatment, lithium intoxication can occur, in which vomiting, diarrhea, tremor, loss of coordination, seizures, and coma can result. Milder forms of this, of course, exist as well. Tremor can be seen even at borderline doses.

Patients on lithium often drink large quantities of water because of an insatiable thirst. This can disturb the fluid and salt balance. Kidney function can also become impaired during lithium treatment, and for this reason, the function of the kidneys should be tested periodically.

Other side effects that can occur even with therapeutic levels of lithium are thyroid disease, allergic reactions, and weight gain. We rarely use lithium as a treatment for migraine.

In addition to the tremor associated with lithium, even at borderline-elevated levels, the person may experience a constant feeling of restlessness. Because this distresses many patients, physicians need to discuss it with them. Again, patient education is essential prior to starting this medication.

Valproic Acid

Valproic acid (Depakene and Depakote) is a relative newcomer in the treatment of migraine. In the past, this medication has been used primarily for various types of epileptic seizures.

Available only orally, valproic acid can cause liver dysfunction, especially in younger individuals, thus should be avoided in patients with a history of compromised liver function. It is often necessary to check blood levels periodically.

Fairly common side effects of this medication are sedation, tremor, and loss of coordination. Other common side effects are loss of appetite, nausea, and vomiting. More rare side effects are allergy, hair loss, and weight gain.

A recent study in Denmark of forty-three patients with migraine revealed that about 50 percent of the patients responded to this therapy. Unfortunately, only the frequency of the migraine responded, while the severity and duration remained unchanged.

Other Medications

Other anti-seizure medications are sometimes used in migraine prevention, such as phenytoin (Dilantin) and carbamazepine (Tegretol). Clonidine has also been thought to play a role in migraine prevention, although recent studies have suggested that this is probably not a good preventive medication.

Some patients report success with various herbs or homeopathic preparations. (See chapter 11 for further information.) It's important, however, that patients who suffer from migraines be under the care of a physician. It's also very important to report all medications that you take to your doctor. They still "count" even if they are Tylenol or a homeopathic remedy you bought in the pharmacy or health food store. Failing to provide your doctor such information could be dangerous for you.

Can My Medications Harm Me?

Medication therapy is quite helpful in treating migraine. In fact, the major advances related to migraine have been pharmacologic. In addition, most people who suffer from severe migraine attacks will at some point benefit from medication. However, certain medications over the long term can be harmful or even cause migraines.

Too Much of Anything Is Bad

Any medication can have side effects that can cause the patient discomfort, disability, and possibly death. For example, acetaminophen (Tylenol) has long been promoted as the ultimate in drug safety. However, as the studies described below indicate, even this over-the-counter medication can have serious side effects and should be used only as prescribed and as infrequently as possible.

It has been known since the 1950s that pain-relieving medications can cause severe kidney damage. In fact, one medication, phenacetin, has clearly been shown to be responsible for kidney failure in many individuals using that medication. What is far less well known is that the main metabolite (breakdown product) of Tylenol is phenacetin.

A recent study in the *New England Journal of Medicine* by Thomas V. Perneger and others gives some reason for alarm for those using large amounts of Tylenol. This powerful study provides fairly convincing statistical arguments discouraging use of this medication on a habitual basis.

In this recent study, 716 patients with chronic renal (kidney) failure were interviewed and compared to 361 age-matched controls without kidney failure. Self-estimates of the amount of consumption of Tylenol, aspirin, and nonsteroidal anti-inflammatory medications were obtained. While there was no suggestion of increased incidents of kidney failure in those taking aspirin, there was evidence of hazards related to Tylenol and nonsteroidal anti-inflammatory medications. The study suggested an increased risk of kidney failure for those taking up to five thousand pills of nonsteroidal anti-inflammatory medications over the course of their lifetime. With regard to Tylenol, a daily consumption of more than one pill per day doubled the odds of chronic renal failure, as did a lifetime consumption of one thousand pills or more.

It should be likewise noted that the risk of drug-related renal failure is increased in persons with diabetes, advanced age, as well as people with problems of dehydration—a frequent consequence of migraine.

The authors of this study proceed with a dramatic suggestion: By reducing the overall consumption of acetaminophen in the population, the number of chronic renal failure cases might be lowered by eight to ten percent. They suggest furthermore that the U.S. could save $500 million to $700 million in estimated care for these patients with chronic renal failure.

Another recent study reported in the *Journals of American Medical Association* by David C. Whitcomb and others identified further risks for the chronic user of acetaminophen. This study was based on the analysis of 49 patients with acetaminophen-related liver injury. Note: It must be emphasized that all these cases were examples of patients taking more than the recommended maximum dose of four grams daily.

Fasting was a potent risk factor in those taking four to ten grams, while recent alcohol use was identified as a risk factor for those taking more than ten grams on a daily basis.

This study has particular relevance with regard to migraine sufferers, as these patients often take more than the intended amount of this medication and often do this unwittingly. They are often unaware that the combination of medications they are taking contain large amounts of Tylenol. Furthermore, the nature of an acute migraine attack, such as severe nausea, vomiting, and inability to eat, essentially represents an unplanned fasting state.

We don't wish to selectively attack acetaminophen and recognize that patients who experienced these side effects may have fared much worse on other medications. We use acetaminophen on a frequent basis in our patients. The point is, however, that we urge our patients to use it as directed and on an intermittent basis. It can be very harmful to assume that a medication that is sold over the counter is automatically "safe."

At this point, we have potent and effective means for treating migraine. But these therapeutic regimens often are a two-edged sword. The information we've included in this chapter should encourage migraineurs to rely as little as possible on medications for their treatment.

To illustrate how a medication that routinely provides excellent pain relief may also play a role in producing a significant problem, the following case illustration is provided:

Complaint: "Migraines"

This 33-year-old right-handed female has a history of headaches associated with nausea, vomiting, and weight loss, dating back to approximately age five. After two or three years, when she was age 8 or 9, the headaches resolved until they returned when she was 26. She had seen three separate eye doctors, who attributed her headache pain to astigmatism.

She described her headaches as involving the whole head, associated with a "funny sound" in her ears, as well as pressure around the skull. They were initially left-sided, but over a two-year evolution, began to involve the entire head. The patient has found that only emergency room visits for narcotics, sleep medication, and indeed, the initiation of sleep are helpful for her pain.

The patient has had an extensive list of medications, including anti-inflammatory medications, muscle relaxers, sleep medicines, pain pills, and strong narcotics. Despite all this, she has continued to experience pain. The patient also sought psychiatric care, as she was concerned that there was a psychiatric component, although this has not been borne out. She has seen prior neurologists, has undergone magnetic imaging of the brain, and on two separate occasions was told that these studies were normal. She has had brain wave scans, again reported as normal.

The patient's history is complicated by an irritable bowel, and by difficulty in tolerating medications. She has a history of mild asthma, kidney stones, and "blackouts" that occurred when she was pregnant. The patient had been placed on numerous medications on a trial basis. Interestingly, she found that the medication Fioricet was quite helpful.

The history becomes quite interesting, in that without any type of narcotic abuse or excess, the patient ended up in the emergency room for drug intoxication. Unfortunately, she was labeled there as a "drug-seeking patient," and was given relatively quick attention. The patient clearly was minimally responsive, lethargic, and barely arousable. Her medication bottles were checked, and she was not taking the medication any more frequently than two or three tablets per day.

She was admitted to the hospital, given intravenous fluids, and after two days, was much improved. Apparently an erratic absorption of the Fioricet from her body's fat tissues led to too much medication in her blood stream and subsequently to her unintentional drug intoxication or "overdose." This was a significant negative reaction to a medication that she was using as directed.

Conclusion

Many types of medications can be tried by your physician. The key is for you to work with a good doctor and cooperate as a team to get rid of—or at least cut back on—the frequency and severity of your migraines. We hope that the information presented in this chapter will further motivate and educate patients to assume responsibility for their care.

11

Non-Pharmacologic Treatments to Control Migraine

S o far in this book, we have discussed what a migraine is in general, what the different categories of headache disorders are, as well as the key mechanisms for producing migraine headaches. We've also talked about the routine treatments and medications prescribed by physicians (especially neurologists) for the treatment of migraine. But we are still left with one fundamental question: "What can I do without seeing my doctor to help control my own migraine headaches?"

This is no trivial question, because it is frequently difficult to see a physician before the migraine starts accelerating in its painful intensity. As discussed earlier, emergency room visits are often not satisfying to the patient with a migraine. In addition, the expense and the time away from work and from daily activities make it extremely impractical to rely on a physician every time you are stricken with a migraine headache.

As a result, this chapter is for people who want to take an active role in initiating therapy for their migraines, particularly with regard to treatments unrelated to using prescribed medications. We discuss diathermy, headband therapy, chiropractic care, therapeutic massage, acupuncture, hypnosis, breathing techniques, guided imagery, progressive relaxation, and homeopathic remedies. We also cover the value of sleep to the migraineur.

Note: We presume that you will continue under the care of a competent and skilled physician. Do not presume that any of these described treatments alone is the one true answer. It's also important that you coordinate your treatments with your physician's.

Non-Medication Treatments

Diathermy (Ice/heat)

In our experience, using ice at the base of the skull is particularly effective for the migraineur, especially at the onset of an acute migraine headache. The ice works in several ways: reduces the inflammation, swelling, and muscle spasm and also acts as a local anesthetic.

Ice also decreases the blood flow to different areas, particularly the base of the skull and muscle, thus preventing the spasm and also delaying the release of chemical mediators from the bloodstream. The ice acts as a shortstop to reduce the "cascade effect" often seen with migraine headache symptoms. It is often effective in aborting an acute attack, or, at the least, it works to significantly reduce the pain.

We've had patients explain to us that they obtain better results with ice placed over the sinus regions at the front of the head. We however, believe that the most effective use of ice packs, particularly when a sick headache starts to come on, is at the base of the skull or back of the neck, and, at times, even across the shoulder area.

If ice doesn't work and the attack gets worse or even seems to evolve into a chronic daily headache, or if the migraine persists for over 48 hours, then heat can be a slightly more effective therapy. Patients often notice that a hot shower, heating pad, or warm compress over the head and over the base of the neck can provide pain relief.

Heat works opposite from the way ice works; it allows small blood vessels to open and enables oxygen and nutrients to reach various muscles and thus to aid with the healing process. This is particularly true in the case of the secondary phenomenon of mixed headache or muscle contraction headaches.

Since either ice or heat may work, both should be tried. Of course, if either makes the symptoms worse, then discontinue and try another method described in this chapter.

Headband

A special headache headband designed and marketed by a California physician, Dr. Vijayan, has provided relief to some migraineurs. Vijayan found that, where local pressure and ice packs have failed, an elastic headband secured with velcro, with rubber discs sited to apply pressure to the area of pain, provided excellent headache relief.

The headband method can be used along with pain medication and vasoconstrictor agents (medicines that cause the blood vessels to narrow), although neither is required.

It's not clear how pain relief was obtained, but the headband did work for patients, according to an article reported in the medical journal *Headache*. Most patients, however, needed to keep the headband in place throughout the course of the headache; if they took it off, the headache came back.

This treatment seems to us both safe and effective, with little or no potential for side effects.

Chiropractic Care

This aspect of non-pharmacologic treatment for migraine could actually merit its own separate chapter, although we will provide as much information as possible in this section. We believe strongly in the value of chiropractic care and have in the past cited numerous articles to our patients that documented the efficacy of chiropractic care, manual care, and manipulation therapy as a safe and effective treatment for soft tissue pain, myofascial pain, and joint pain syndromes.

Many patients receive a great deal of pain relief from chiropractic manipulations received on a frequent basis, and some chiropractic physicians will treat patients for not only spinal column dysfunction but also for significant headache symptoms.

Without medication usage and with proper spinal adjustment performed in the hands of a competent and certified chiropractic physician, the treatment can be a very positive experience that produces outstanding pain relief for the patient. It's also important to note that the chiropractic physicians with whom we work are also highly educated on wellness and health education and often provide additional information about the patient's activities that may actually trigger migraine.

Chiropractic care is also highly effective for neck pain syndromes, which can produce daily headaches that are often confused with the chronic migraine. A proper spinal alignment can reduce joint inflammation and instability in the cervical spine and should certainly be considered as one reasonable approach when it comes to non-pharmacologic therapy.

Therapeutic Massage

On many occasions, we have prescribed therapeutic massage intervention to abort an acute migraine attack. Three massage therapists work for us and achieve a high level of success with our patients.

If you do not know a reputable facility that provides massages, ask your physician for a recommendation. Often massage therapy is used in conjunction with diathermy (especially heat) for a combined treatment of about ten to twenty minutes, concentrating on the areas of greatest muscle spasm and muscle tension.

Massage seems to be a three-pronged action mechanism, and any one of the three factors may be the one to reduce headache pain; however, we feel that a combination of these mechanisms brings about a positive outcome.

First, therapeutic massage is inherently relaxing for patients. By simply presenting themselves for a massage, myofascial release, and manipulative care, our patients are removing themselves from their routine environment and placing themselves into a non-stressful, often dark, and quite peaceful environment. This change alone has positive effects, not only in removing possible headache triggers but also in allowing patients to reframe their environment.

Second, the preparation for therapeutic massage and the act of receiving massage can usually be relaxing and reduce stress and anxiety. As anyone who has suffered a severe migraine headache can testify, one major problem that occurs when a migraine symptom first presents is the acute anxiety associated with the headache.

Anxiety-escalating questions—"Oh, no! Am I going to get sick? Will I have to leave work? Will I have to stop what I'm doing?"—are almost inevitable for many migraine sufferers.

This anxiety can then lead to a rebound phenomenon, with the associated release of additional stress chemicals (catecholamines) and the building up of toxins and waste products, which often result from muscle contraction, muscle spasm, and tissue breakdown products such as lactic acid.

All these factors taken together contribute to produce additional aggravation of the headache pain. But by reducing the anxiety, on the other hand, one can also reduce the adrenaline and stress chemicals that are often associated with anxiety. This in turn often leads to a reduction in pain and certainly can also reduce the severity and duration of the headache.

The final, and possibly the most effective, mechanism of action in therapeutic massage is the physical trigger release, myofascial release, and the direct muscle anti-inflammatory effect of the massage itself.

The actual massage can break down tissue triggers that are also frequently seen in both migraine and chronic daily headache sufferers. In addition, we often also see improved flexibility and range of motion, and decreased spasm and muscle triggers (mini-spasms in the muscle) in direct response to the therapeutic massage.

A total body massage often helps the person to relax, reduces stress chemicals, and improves the overall sensation of wellness. Conversely, a focal massage over the neck and shoulder region can aid to reduce local triggers, and thereby enable other body muscles to relax. As a result, muscle tightening throughout the body is avoided.

Remember that just as an open communication with your physician is essential to your continued good health, so is an open communication with your massage therapist. If there are techniques, procedures, or any aspects of the therapy that seem to cause an increased discomfort or irritation of your muscles, be sure to tell the therapist. Operate with your therapist as a team. Be assertive.

Also, don't assume that if one massage therapist or therapy technique fails to provide relief, then massage therapy can't work for you. Instead, explore different options with your therapist. Ask what type of therapy he or she prefers to do, or try another therapist.

Acupuncture

Although some doctors refuse to believe that nontraditional therapeutic interventions can play a positive role in pain relief, we, on the other hand, have seen therapeutic benefits with acupuncture intervention.

Acupuncture, an ancient Eastern treatment, can lead to a release of the body's own pain messengers—endorphins and enkephalins. These are our own personal morphine and opi-ate-like substances, which are released by the body when we have pain. (These are also released by long-distance runners during a race, allowing them to experience the euphoria of the marathon run.)

Researchers don't know how acupuncture works, although some research has revealed that if a patient is given a chemical that blocks morphine (such as naloxone or natrexone), then the chemical also appears to completely block the effects of acupuncture therapy. This means that the body's own pain chemicals were either (a) not released or (b) the chemical receptors they are trying to act upon are saturated with the blocking medicines.

Eastern medicine has used acupuncture for many years to provide pain relief and pain blocking. In some cases, acupuncture has even been used to block pain during surgical procedures.

Acupuncture may also affect the gastrointestinal (stom-ach and intestine) system. As discussed earlier in the book, there is a slowing of the bowel and stomach function during the onset of acute migraine; the stomach may become nearly paralyzed. Acupuncture seems to overcome this "gastro-paresis" thus leading to a significant reduction in the nausea of the migraine headache.

Hypnosis

Hypnosis is a state of mind that can lead to pain reduction or even pain elimination. It is difficult to initiate when the patient is in the middle of an agonizing migraine attack. However, patients can be trained to self-hypnotize and mod-ify their own behavior and habits and even to control their body temperatures.

Once patients have been trained in hypnotherapy, they may be able to abort their headache with hypnosis when they feel a migraine coming on.

Hypnosis is a form of extremely focused attention, which, when effective, can shift the focus away from the migraine pain syndrome. In addition, if the patient can alter the body temperature, this is another effective means of controlling pain, just as is diathermy. In effect, you are icing or heating yourself with your own brain and nothing else.

Hypnotherapy is clearly a learned skill and one that needs to be practiced frequently by the patient, in both the pain and pain-free state.

Breathing Techniques

If you're alive, you know how to breathe correctly, right? Wrong! Proper breathing is actually a function that we take for granted. But during the onset of an acute migraine, a patient often has accelerated breathing patterns and shallow respirations. Breathing incorrectly can then reinforce the pain syndrome—not something you want to happen!

The nervous system regulates your heart rate, pulse, breathing, and so on. And there is a feedback mechanism through which our breathing systems can send either correct or incorrect signals back to the nervous system. Through this route, we can change and improve our central nervous system.

If we breathe correctly, we can send correct messages back to the brain; therefore, we have a chance to alter the outflow of improper messages through this feedback loop. As a result, we slow the migraine cascade, which ultimately leads to a blockade of at least a portion of the migraine syndrome.

How do you breathe correctly? During an acute attack, chemical messengers are released in the brain. One key messenger is adrenaline, our stress chemical that produces the reactive feeling of "fight or flight."

As a result of adrenaline release, we then have rapid shallow breathing and often use the diaphragm (site of the main muscles for breathing) as well as other accessory muscles.

Using these additional muscles can cause muscle tightness and contraction of the neck and shoulder muscles. This in turn leads to reinforcement of improper breathing as well as to breakdown products—toxins that ultimately circulate in the bloodstream.

To correct and even reverse this pathological response to pain, we must focus and concentrate on achieving proper breathing techniques. Breathing from the diaphragm allows you to focus on your stomach muscles and move the diaphragm in a slow and controlled breathing. As with hypnotherapy, diaphragmatic breathing (or deep breathing) exercises are usually best performed in a calm, comfortable, and quiet environment. Therefore, it's a good idea to practice your breathing exercises while well and not in the grip of an acute migraine attack.

Breathe slowly and steadily, with a deep inhale and slow exhale, while concentrating on your abdominal muscles. Some physicians also supplement deep breathing with biofeedback, temperature measurements, and muscle skin sensitivity readings. We prefer to allow our patients to breathe at a regular and steady pace, finding the cadence and rhythm that works best for them.

Once patients are comfortable with these breathing techniques, they should perform them immediately upon the onset of any prodrome or any premonition of a sick headache coming on. Deep breathing is positive protocol to follow on a regular basis. Set aside two to three minutes, three or four times each day, for this simple exercise as a preventive measure for migraine and daily headaches.

Guided Imagery

Another form of a relaxation technique is guided imagery. This involves attempting to elicit a response by visualizing a positive image, with the goal of triggering a reaction from the brain. Guided imagery may take the form of imagining yourself floating, seeing yourself in a calm environment, or imagining yourself in a safe, protected environment.

The more focused you can be and the more detailed the vision in your mind, the more positive a response you can obtain. Practitioners of guided imagery and hypnosis will often use both to elicit the same response—to trigger a beneficial nervous system response.

Guided imagery, like hypnosis, should be practiced, preferably during a healthy pain-free period.

Progressive Relaxation

Progressive relaxation is a simple technique that is easy to start and do, even for a novice. This technique deals with contracting and relaxing individual muscles. In your mind, you may start with the toes and feet, working your way up to the calves, thighs, buttocks, then to the trunk, hands and arms, shoulders, and finally the neck and scalp. You should focus intensely on each muscle involved, contracting it for ten to twenty seconds and then relaxing it for thirty to sixty seconds.

This technique will not provide immediate relief but often can shift the focus away from a migraine attack and onto the individual muscles that you are progressively relaxing. You try to "fool the nervous system" into thinking that it does not need to pay attention to the migraine chemical pattern that is occurring.

Sleep and Natural Sleep Inducers

Most migraineurs know that lying down in a dark and quiet room, removing triggers, and, most importantly, falling asleep, can be an effective treatment for the acute migraine attack. Sleep has been noted in numerous journals and treatment plans as a key treatment of choice for the pain management of an acute migraine.

One theory of sleep as a treatment for migraine is that it allows the brain to "reset itself," somewhat like resetting a computer. As the migraine chemicals are dumped throughout the brain, sleep is a restorative process, which seems to allow an appropriate re-uptake of this flood of chemicals. As a result, the brain can re-regulate itself and allow only the proper flow of chemicals.

While this is a theory rather than proven fact, it makes sense. Virtually all migraine sufferers have noticed that falling asleep then waking up later is a partial, if not complete, treatment of severe migraine headaches. If you can fall asleep without medication, fine. But we think it is also important to mention that there are over-the-counter treatments for sleep initiation.

One of the best we've seen is melatonin, a natural chemical. There is talk that the Federal Drug Administration (FDA) may make melatonin a controlled substance, but at the present time, it is a safe and effective therapy that often produces sleep without that groggy, hung-over effect upon awakening. Melatonin is not a sedative nor is it habit-forming or addictive.

Homeopathic Medications and Remedies

Today in many pharmacies you can find homeopathic medications sold without a prescription. Are they any good?

We are not experts or specialists in homeopathic health care, but we are asked frequently about natural medications and natural treatment regimens. We are "allopathic" (traditional) physicians; however, we believe some important comments should be made about homeopathic remedies.

Homeopathy, a discipline of nontraditional medicine was founded by German physician Dr. Samuel Christian Friedrich Hahnemann in the late eighteenth century. Its premise is that if large doses of medicines or substances produce certain symptoms, then small doses of the same substance can cure those symptoms. Having been around for over a hundred years, homeopathy clearly has a significant place in providing comfort and pain management for many migraine sufferers. It is quite popular in other countries and is emerging slowly in the United States.

We often like to explain to our patients that it is best to have many "tricks in your bag," and if one therapy does not work, at least there are many more to try. We believe that if we were only to have a hammer in our arsenal of tools, then the world would look like a series of nails and nothing else. That clearly is not the case. So, the point is that there is some room for homeopathy—although the size of that role is not yet clear.

How does homeopathic medicine work—if it does work? One theory is that minute doses of a substance that would be harmful in large doses can stimulate healing in the body. For example, belladonna is a deadly poison if a large enough dose is taken, but very small doses may cure your migraine. Homeopathic medicine may allow the body to heal itself by "resetting" the body's imbalances that led to the migraine headache. How it does this remains a mystery.

A variety of chemicals or medications are popular among homeopathic physicians. Each one appears to direct its action against specific symptoms. Do remember that patients respond differently to different medications, and this is also true with homeopathic medicine.

As a result, it is important to practice a trial-and-error approach to homeopathic medicines (under the guidance of an expert), just as it is important to use this approach with traditional medicines. Belladonna seems to be effective for patients who have severe intractable headaches that are associated with throbbing blood vessels and facial flushing, as well as with headaches aggravated by standing and improved by sitting down.

Bryonia seems to work with motion-sensitive headaches, as well as headaches associated with moderate pain behind the eyes. In addition, migraines that are present in the early morning, particularly upon awakening, may respond to bryonia. If you feel sinus congestion or fullness, you may have a positive response to this chemical.

Nux vomica is another homeopathic remedy. You may improve with this substance if your migraines appear to be induced by eating or drinking—for example, if consuming coffee or caffeine-full substances brings on a migraine. In addition, if you've had basic changes to your schedule, such as sleep, nutrition, diet, or activity-level changes that trigger your migraine, you may respond to this medication.

Pulsatilla is a substance that may help you if you suffer from the "brain freeze" of eating a cold substance that triggers a migraine. If smoking or over-indulging in rich foods causes your migraine, you may also respond to this medication.

Geisemium is another homeopathic remedy; it seems most effective if your headache syndrome begins at the back of your neck then radiates forward. Headaches associated with visual aura may also respond to this treatment.

Sanguinaria is a homeopathic remedy for patients who suffer from migraine pain on one side of the head. Also, intractable headaches, without pounding and throbbing, may respond to this medication.

Some herbs may also be used to treat migraine headaches. For example, feverfew seems fairly effective for some patients as a preventive measure to avoid the acute migraine episode. Articles reviewed by the National Headache Foundation have stated that it is somewhat effective for migraine prevention. Apparently this herb must be taken on a regular basis. However, it should be noted that the use of feverfew is still considered an experimental therapy among traditional neurologists. Large controlled studies have yet to be performed using feverfew compared to prescription medications.

Readers interested in more information about homeopathic medications, remedies, and treatments should do a more extensive review of the available literature. You'll get a head start by referring to the sources and treatment options listed in the bibliography and appendix.

12

Taking Control—
Lifestyle Changes

Up to this point, we have discussed migraine and other types of headaches, multiple facets relating to migraine disorders, and how physicians approach issues relating to diagnosing and treating migraineurs. Now we will focus on how *you* can take control of your activities and other aspects of your life to work toward preventing migraines from occurring, or at least minimizing the pain they cause. The following suggestions can also improve your overall physical functioning.

Getting Your Body into a Healthy Cycle

Our bodies are complex machines, and just like other complicated pieces of equipment, they cannot be run 24 hours a day without some "down time." Also like intricate equipment, we need frequent maintenance and periodic checkups.

Most importantly of all, we function most efficiently when we are on a basic routine. The body works on a chemical routine, particularly with relation to the peaks and valleys related to the adrenaline chemicals that are produced. We have peaks of cortisol, an adrenaline chemical, at approximately 6:00 A.M. and 4:00 P.M. This may explain why we start out the day with energy, by early to mid-afternoon have periods of fatigue, then in late afternoon get a "second wind."

When we try to break this cycle or resist our bodies' natural rhythm, we can end up experiencing a general sense of fatigue, malaise, and being unwell. As mentioned previously, any illness and any competition with our bodies' natural rhythms can certainly act as a migraine or headache trigger. Therefore, it is best to pick a routine and try to regiment our lifestyle enough so that we can live comfortably within the boundaries of our routine.

This is not to say that we expect our readers to become robots with a rigidly restricted lifestyle, looking at the clock every hour to maintain their regimen. Rather, we recommend that you try to wake up at the same time every morning and eat three to four small, well-balanced meals per day. Space out work and exercise, as well as your social obligations and stressful activities, in a pattern comfortable for you.

We know this can't always be done. Maybe your mother-in-law or boss is coming for dinner, the kids just came down with chicken pox, and you're also juggling a difficult project—so for today you have to throw out most of your schedule. These things happen. But within the parameters of your life, you do have quite a bit of control (yes, you do!), and we want you to use it.

Everyone needs to examine his or her lifestyle to determine what the daily priorities are and to then determine how those can be broken up. One of the common factors in patients who experience migraines when they travel is the fact that they are not only having altitude and geographic changes, but also changes to their daily routine. We frequently hear "My whole vacation was ruined by my migraine headaches."

Part of this is because you may be consuming foods different from your usual diet. But a bigger part of the problem is that you may get yourself completely out of sync; for example, a time zone change can throw you off because it affects your sleeping and eating patterns, and there also may be climactic and altitude changes, as well as other differences from your normal life.

We recommend to our patients that even when they travel, they try to maintain a routine lifestyle, or at least as close to a routine lifestyle as possible.

Pearl of wisdom: As we mentioned earlier in this chapter, our cortisol level drops early in the afternoon, and doesn't pick up again until late afternoon. This may explain why most country's citizens (with the notable exception of people in the United States) take naps or respite periods after lunchtime.

Although you may not be able to take an afternoon nap, it may still be a good idea to avoid over-exerting yourself in the mid-afternoon, particularly if you are prone to peaks and valleys of adrenaline chemicals in your body.

Sleep Better, Live Better

Following through on this concept of a routine lifestyle, we certainly cannot ignore what for most people is approximately one-third of their life—sleep time. We have often heard the expression, "If I could just get a good night's sleep, I know I would feel better." This is absolutely true. Sleep is an important physiological function that acts to restore the body's nutrients and indeed allows us to "re-set the computer."

When we have difficulties with sleep initiation (insomnia), as well as difficulties with staying asleep or waking up too early, we often do not fully recharge our bodies. In this sense, we're much like a nickel cadmium rechargeable battery. If the body is not drained down completely, then when it is charged, the charge does not last as long. Certainly, if we do not get a full complement or battery of sleep, when we do awaken, we are rarely as refreshed or energetic as we would like to be, nor do we "last as long" without becoming fatigued and sleepy.

The American Sleep Disorders Foundation has eloquently stated that many actually acquire a "sleep debt." People will go for days or even weeks getting too little sleep and then have to spend a few days actually replacing that sleep debt with a long weekend of extended sleep pattern.

Certainly, this extreme variation in the day/night cycle, and in the body's natural rhythms, can lead to discomfort and can even be a potent trigger for illness, including migraines.

Correcting the Sleep Problem

It is clear that before we can correct the sleep problem, one needs to identify what is actually causing the sleep disturbance. For many individuals, it is the chemicals that they ingest, but for others it is lifestyle stressors, inappropriate activities, or simply an uncomfortable sleeping environment.

Indeed, one of the most notorious triggers for insomnia is actually sleep medications. While they may work for a series of days, they frequently lead to a rebound phenomenon, a secondary insomnia, which is quite difficult to treat.

Specialists who deal with sleep disorders often recommend a comprehensive sleep evaluation, even going so far as monitoring someone's sleep in a laboratory at nighttime. If there is a reversal of one's day/night cycle, or if someone is off by "two or three hours" after traveling, many techniques can be used to "re-set your time clock"; however, these are not trivial and are best discussed with a specialist in sleep disorders.

To correct a problematic sleep cycle, follow these simple rules:

- Do not consume any caffeine or stimulant medication close to bedtime. Many authorities would recommend avoiding caffeine entirely at any time, particularly if there is any sleep problem, and certainly if caffeine is a headache trigger for you.

- Avoid alcoholic beverages prior to bedtime. The idea of "just a nightcap will help me fall asleep" may be correct, but almost assuredly will wake you up within a few hours.

Actually, alcohol does three things to the central nervous system: irritates, inflames, and depresses. So while alcohol may act as a central nervous system depressant initially, there is a profound rebound effect that occurs within two to three hours and also acts as a rebound stimulant.

This is why individuals who imbibe alcoholic beverages in mid-evening can often be drowsy throughout the night but later on are "wide awake and ready to keep going."

- If you cannot sleep, it is absolutely essential that you get up, get out of bed, and do something else. Do not lie in bed and wait for sleep to come; oftentimes it will not, and trying to sleep just leads to a frustration or anxiety situation, which then leads to additional sleep dysfunction.
- Avoid re-setting the "sleep clock" by taking little naps throughout the course of the day. We do allow some of our senior citizens to take a one-half to one-hour nap after lunch, when the cortisol levels are low, but this would be only if their naps do not compromise their sleep habits (i.e., keep them up later than usual). With regard to our migraine sufferers, we absolutely do not want them to interrupt their day cycle with sleep, as that will also interrupt their night cycle with wakefulness.
- Do not go to bed angry or stressed. While this sounds simple, it is surprising how many people will truly "take their problems to bed," and then simply rehash them all night. They toss and turn, which clearly is unhealthy.

We explain to our patients that it is very important they resolve their crises, problems, or dilemmas prior to sleep. Yes, we know this is easy to say, hard to do. But try it! It has worked for many. Despite sounding simple and trivial, our patients have told us that when they do follow this instruction, they have a much more restful night of sleep.

Now that we have discussed what not to do, we can be more positive by pointing out actions that are helpful when you want to fall to sleep.

- Work on, practice, and develop positive relaxation techniques to initiate drowsiness and restfulness.

- Be assertive—prepare your sleep environment to make it comfortable for you. Specifically, eliminate activity, noises, sounds, or lights that keep you awake. Many individuals tell us that with "white noise," or soothing background noise, they can effectively block out irritating noise.

- Check with your doctor and check with your pharmacist for guidance. Frequently, even medications that have been taken for a long period of time, or medicines that your physician has told you "won't have any side effects," may in fact have a stimulant effect. It is important to check on this, as there is almost always more than one medication for any one illness.

Don't be afraid to communicate with your physician that this disruption in your sleep cycle is an issue. It certainly is an issue when you suffer from migraine headache disorder.

In addition to those general concepts for preparing for a proper sleep cycle, some more specific suggestions are often helpful. For example, L-tryptophan, an amino acid, has been noted to be quite helpful for sleep initiation. This drug was recently banned from the United States, but is once again available here as well as in other countries. However, there are also many natural methods of obtaining L-tryptophan.

Foods high in L-tryptophan content include such things as bananas, yogurt, dates, and milk. (See? Your mom was right if she told you to drink a nice glass of milk before bed!)

In addition, certain vitamins and supplements have also been found somewhat helpful in improving sleep initiation, such as Vitamin B3, as well as calcium and magnesium. Indeed, numerous investigations currently underway have revealed that magnesium is a potent mineral and may play an extremely important role in aborting acute migraine headaches.

Also, many herbs are helpful for sleep initiation, such as valerian root and passion flower.

Leg Cramp Problems

We are frequently questioned about nighttime leg cramps, which often awaken patients from sleep and seem to prevent the re-initiation of sleep. Prescription medications such as quinine sulfate and Quinam can help alleviate this problem. But a more natural approach can include such simple measures as good relaxation techniques prior to bed, as well as taking Vitamin E supplements. We have had quite good results with this.

Natural Sleep Substance

Lastly, a natural hormone, melatonin, reaches its peak of activity during sleep. Produced in the pineal gland, melatonin seems to play a powerful role in maintaining a regular hormonal and circadian cycle (a daily fluctuation of hormone release and other physiological functions). At the present time, prescription melatonin is not widely available. For more information regarding how to obtain this chemical, you should consult your physician.

Exercise

If you look around at the newspaper, on television, or at your local bookstore, you will gain the impression that exercise is a cure for everything, or at least that seems to be what people want you to believe. And they are probably right. Not only does exercise help you look good, it actually enables you to feel good and be well.

A number of processes occur with routine exercise, such as increasing your metabolism, burning fat, reducing calories, and improving your cardiovascular system. For patients suffering from migraine disorders, routine exercise can actually produce complex chemical changes in the brain that may ward off future migraine attacks.

We have one patient who tells us that when he gets his migraine headaches, he will actually "go for a jog" to try to avoid a severe attack from coming on. Often his migraine episode is completely aborted within 5–10 minutes, without any of the severe nausea or secondary phenomenon.

How does this work? Well, we think that the exercise-induced chemical change induces a blockade of chemical response, thereby preventing the blood vessels going in and out of spasm, and reducing the ultimate pounding, throbbing, and pulsing headache pain.

To provide an example, the exercise produces chemical messengers that act sort of as a key fitting into the lock. When these chemical messengers (the good guys) fit in the lock, that means that the poisons or toxins that occur at the time of a migraine headache cannot fit into this same "lock."

Therefore, the whole cascade effect (discussed in chapter 2: Theories of Migraine) cannot occur, and we are "protected." While exercise does not produce this effect in every individual, certainly it has many benefits for virtually everyone.

We often recommend that patients do a combination of exercise, not just body toning or just aerobic activity. We combine a low-impact aerobic program with a weight or resistance training program, in combination with proper body mechanics (to be discussed later).

We generally recommend 30–40 minutes of aerobic activities three to four times per week plus a resistance training program with low weights and multiple repetitions three to four times a week for 30–40 minutes each.

We know what you are thinking—we've heard it before. "But Doctor, I don't *have* 60 to 80 minutes a day to exercise!" However, when you think about it, if you provide yourself with positive reinforcement and positive conditioning by training for approximately one hour per day, that still leaves 23 hours in your whole day. This seems a pretty reasonable balance when you consider that the return can be a pain-free existence.

Nutrition: "You Are What You Eat"

Most of us have automobiles or often ride in automobiles. If you have ever obtained bad gasoline, you know what the effect can be. Your car does not run well, and ultimately you suffer for it. The initial savings the cheaper gasoline may have offered is far outweighed by the frustration, annoyance, and ultimately larger costs one has to pay down the road.

Our bodies also require good fuel to run well. While neither of us is extremist about diet or habits, we do promote the values of moderation, particularly when it comes to a proper diet. And for migraine sufferers, a proper diet can be everything.

In the 1960s, the rage was for neurologists to place patients on what is called an "oligo-antigenic diet." This is a special type of elimination diet. It allows the dieter to pinpoint what foods may be migraine triggers by introducing food back into the diet one type at a time. We have come a long way since this diet, yet as we have discussed in our chapter on food fright, diet is still absolutely essential in managing the migraine headache.

It isn't possible to know every ingredient in each food, but certainly reading labels is appropriate, as is avoiding toxins such as caffeine (found in beverages such as coffee, tea, and colas as well as foods made from cocoa), avoiding processed foods high in sulfites or MSG, and staying away from foods containing excessive yeast, nitrates/nitrites, or tyramine.

Although a glass of milk may help you get to sleep, for some migraineurs, dairy products can have a negative impact. This fact is certainly outlined in the National Headache Foundation's Diet, as well as in numerous additional diets for migraine patients.

So what type of diet is an appropriate diet to prevent or control migraine attacks? Experts disagree, but we feel the key is moderation. While in some instances it is a good idea to go to a complete elimination diet, introducing one food at a time, it certainly is reasonable to cut down on foods high in cholesterol, fat, and sugar content.

In addition, too much red meat may act as a food trigger, thus your intake of red meat certainly should be reduced. Since red meat is predominantly made up of fat and protein, too much red meat may in turn lead to a high protein count, which then has to be metabolized. Physicians have already found that in certain illnesses such as liver and kidney disease, as well as in neurologic illness such as Parkinson's, a low-protein diet can be very effective in controlling them. Certainly, many theories regarding low-protein diets have also been hypothesized for migraine disorders.

In addition, it is reasonable to consider a routine daily multivitamin/multimineral supplement. However, we urge you away from a mega-vitamin preparation. In addition, avoid the "amino acid therapy," which we see many of today's teens using, particularly teenage athletes.

There are good vitamins that are effective as anti-oxidants, a topic which certainly has received some popular press over the last few years. Such chemicals include Vitamins E and C, selenium, and even beta-carotene. You can go to any health food store and find a wide variety and complement of combinations of these antioxidants, as well as of vitamin and mineral supplements. (The Life Guide Diet Supplement, which is listed in the Appendix, is an example of a vitamin preparation.)

When patients come to us with migraine disorders, we ask that they bring all the chemicals and medicines they take, including natural treatments, non-prescription medications, and over-the-counter medications. It is surprising what patients will take in the name of "natural herbs and supplements," just because it does not require a prescription from a physician.

Additional supplements that are often found in good multi-vitamin/multimineral supplements include chromium, copper, iron, manganese, molybdenum, potassium, and zinc.

Key Supplements

While Vitamin B6 (pyridoxine) may not be the one essential ingredient for a neurochemical process, it is now recognized as a powerful cofactor for almost every neurologic chemical process that occurs in the body.

Specifically, one can think of B6 as a taxi driver for additional chemicals and nutrients. B6 helps the chemicals and nutrients get where they need to be, but does not actually participate in the chemical reaction once these materials reach their destination.

Much like the taxi driver, B6 is a cofactor and is extremely important. In neurology, we see B6 deficiency producing seizures, particularly in children and newborn infants. A B6 deficiency also plays a significant role in headache disorder, particularly vascular headaches.

Other complications of B6 deficiency include neuropathy (nerve damage in the extremities), behavior change, mood swings, depression, and even movement disorders. B6 deficiency can actually have a significant role in perpetuating a chronic pain syndrome.

In addition, a subset of migraine exists that occurs with the chemical and hormonal shifts associated with premenstrual syndrome, which is quite well addressed with a combined effect of pyridoxine (B6) and magnesium.

As mentioned, B6 seems to be an important chemical link for many chemical reactions in the body, particularly as the "express taxi driver" for magnesium. Recently magnesium has received a lot of attention with regard to numerous medical processes, including providing significant relief for migraine headaches.

Magnesium

While we are talking about supplements, we should spend a moment discussing the positive breakthroughs with regard to understanding the role of magnesium. We now know that a lack of magnesium in the diet can lead to deficiencies, but we also know that other medical illnesses, including sugar diabetes, thyroid disease, and multiple medications, can lead to this deficiency of magnesium as well.

Alcohol and prolonged stress can also be factors in a low magnesium level. In addition to triggering a migraine headache or promoting a migraine into a severe sick headache, symptoms of low magnesium can include muscle cramps, general fatigue, sleep disturbance, irritability, and muscle tension.

As mentioned earlier, prolonged stress or illness can lead to a magnesium deficiency. Here we see a cyclical pattern, that the low magnesium level leads to illness, and the illness continues the low magnesium level by depleting magnesium stores.

We recommend to our patients that they have their magnesium levels monitored, and we also recommend that magnesium-deficient patients may increase their magnesium levels through consuming such foods as nuts, beans, whole grains, and fish.

Because the magnesium seems to play a significant role in stabilizing the blood vessel walls, thus preventing the spasm, it is absolutely critical that physicians take a look at magnesium levels. While it is unlikely that magnesium is the sole culprit in causing or allowing a migraine to continue, it is nevertheless an easily and quickly treated problem, and therefore should be addressed and remedied.

We strongly recommend that you discuss vitamin deficiencies and whether you should take a general vitamin and mineral supplement with your physician to make sure you are on the right path with regard to overall nutritional wellness. One popular and relatively complete supplement is the Life Guide Adult Daily Dietary Supplement, which can be obtained at many natural health stores. (More information on this supplement is included in the Appendix.)

Herbs and Natural Ingredients

While traditional Western medicine places great stock in the value of prescription medications, it is important to realize that almost every medication has its origins in a natural product, almost always plant products.

Keeping this in mind, you shouldn't be surprised that a natural alternative to prescription medications are herbs, which may be used as medicinal agents. There are literally thousands of these available at the natural health stores, and one has to exercise great judgment and caution in approaching them, just as you should with any over-the-counter medicine or any prescription medicine.

As we tell our patients, any chemical can have any reaction in any one individual, so it is important to make sure that you know what the potential desired effect is, and then monitor for side effects appropriately.

In previous chapters, we have discussed a handful of natural ingredients that are frequently used to treat migraine pain. Another common example is feverfew. This member of the daisy family is believed to work by blocking serotonin release. Also, it possibly inhibits the release of additional chemical substances in the brain that are responsible for causing the spasm in the blood vessel walls. This is an extremely popular chemical remedy in England.

Additional herbal treatments for acute migraine attacks include white willow bark, a compound very similar to aspirin. Also, L-tryptophan used as an amino acid supplement may actually help raise the pain threshold, thereby reducing the appreciation of pain. An additional amino acid, phenylalanine, may actually be able to block the breakdown of the brain's natural pain medicines, endorphins/enkephalins. Endorphins, which are the chemical released to produce the "runner's high" in long distance runners, are much like morphine, and can be used as natural painkillers.

Since literally hundreds of chemicals are available for the natural treatment of pain and migraines, we refer you to our list of resources in the Appendix on where to obtain more information.

Posture

Parents often say: "Sit up straight, keep your back straight, don't slouch." Once again, Mom (or Dad) was right. Posture plays a significant role in maintaining proper spine alignment and preventing the forces of injury, which can lead to muscle spasm and muscle contraction. As we have discussed, there are multiple theories of migraine, yet the brain itself does not appreciate pain. There are no pain-sensitive structures in the brain. We experience pain from either involvement of the arteries and small arterioles, or from the sensation triggers in the neck, head, and joints.

When we slouch, stoop forward, hold our head in one isolated posture for prolonged periods of time, we have improper forces applied to the cervical musculature, and with this there is tension and stress on the supporting structures of the head and neck. This then leads to spasm, waste products from the spasm, including toxins, and ultimately, spasm of the blood vessels. Along with these actions, there is also a decreased circulation, decreased oxygen and nutrition, and ultimately, we experience pain.

We recommend that our patients follow proper body mechanics (please see neck exercises in the Appendix) and make frequent changes in position. Don't keep your head or neck in any isolated posture for more than 40–45 minutes at a time without a 3–5 minute change in position.

While this may sound like a significant time commitment, especially in a work environment with close supervision, one can take a 3–5 minute change in position by changing from the computer to do filing, from filing to walking to the water cooler or copier, and so on. As a result, we don't mean that you have to put a screeching halt to all activity every 45 minutes. It merely means you should change positions.

It's also important to note that individuals who follow a routine exercise regimen, utilize proper body mechanics, and demonstrate good posture, rarely will have the secondary muscle contraction phenomenon that seems to plague many migraine sufferers. Migraineurs may develop a mixed headache disorder, having both migraines and their daily headache pains, which are not true migraines. Because proper body posture can eliminate secondary muscle contraction, we outline key ways to achieve good posture in our Appendix under Activities for Daily Living. Proper stretching and flexibility exercises are also presented.

Deficiency in the "Coping Chromosome"

We all have our own ways to handle both physical and emotional stress. Some people ignore the problem; others tackle it head-on. Some internalize problems, while others verbalize them until everyone knows about their situation. With migraine pain, the most important thing is to enhance your own personal coping mechanisms.

We do not have a "coping chromosome." Instead, we learn through our environment, society, and positive and negative reinforcements on how to deal effectively with stressful situations.

Certainly, recurrent headaches, as well as intractable migraines, can be considered both an external and internal stress. We need to not only alleviate the pain, but improve our outlook and reduce the anxiety that comes with the expectation of pain. We need to regain control of our lives.

But how? One of the first things that we instruct our patients to do is to identify triggers and eliminate these from their environment. Specifically, you are to avoid chemicals, toxins, and body pollutants (tobacco, alcohol, caffeine, etc.) you are currently using. In fact, it is important you remove these triggers from your environment altogether if possible.

If your spouse smokes, make it clear that their smoke may be triggering your headache pains; therefore, this situation needs to be remedied. If your spouse is unable or unwilling to give up smoking, could he or she confine the smoking to an outside area? Can you seek other mutually acceptable solutions?

In addition, make sure you follow a good lifestyle regimen, which includes frequent nutritional meals and avoidance of low sugar (hypoglycemic) states.

How you perceive your pain is another important issue you need to address. If, with the onset of a mild, dull headache you become anxious and your heart races, you become fearful that maybe you'll develop a severe migraine. Often this reaction itself will promote the very reactions you want so badly to avoid.

Using the nonpharmacologic treatments listed in other chapters, you can often immediately perform one or more of these activities (muscle relaxation, deep breathing, guided imagery, etc.) to help block the secondary response to migraine. Yes, a dull headache may present and may progress into a migraine. Yet how we react to this and how we interact immediately plays a significant role in determining what our ultimate level of illness and dysfunction may be.

We have one patient who explained to us that when he feels his headache coming on, he steps into the bathroom and uses an Imitrex injection. He will remain in the toilet stall for approximately 8–12 minutes. The result is that nearly every single sequential event leading up to the migraine has been completely aborted, with the patient able to resume unrestricted work activities. In the meantime, not a single co-employee knew that he had a severe headache/migraine, nor does anyone notice those few minutes away from his work station. As a result, this migraineur has had no negative repercussions, and has been a very successful employee.

Many of our patients have complained of a multitude of psychological symptoms, either directly or indirectly associated with their migraine headaches: fatigue, sadness, depression, crying spells, feelings of emptiness and hopelessness, anxiety, and especially a "generalized or free-floating anxiety." Patients also complain of an overall lack of drive, lack of appetite, decreased attention and concentration, and memory disturbances.

It is essential to be able to identify these sensations as they correlate with migraine headache pain. It is equally critical to take control of these feelings, emotions, and attitudes in order to effect a positive response to your headache treatment, and also to your lifestyle and general sense of wellness.

Sometimes, however, you may need assistance from a mental professional who can help you develop additional coping mechanisms and undergo personal growth counseling. You may need an unbiased, objective listener who can see aspects of your lifestyle or behaviors that you yourself can't see (just as you couldn't see the "Kick Me!" sign another third grader taped to your back) and who can play a role in your recovery. An unbiased professional may be able to determine other triggers, other activities in which you are engaging that somehow may be promoting your migraine headaches. In addition, the mental health professional may be able to identify associated psychological symptoms that come on with the anxiety and stress of a headache syndrome.

As you can see, it is important to follow a complete lifestyle approach to headache pain management, which includes avoidance of inappropriate medication, herbs, or chemicals; replacement of the proper body minerals, nutrients, and vitamin supplements; diet; exercise; and proper body mechanics. A proper sleep and life cycle and a positive outlook can all play a tremendous role in improving your headache syndrome and alleviating your migraine dysfunction.

Remember, the migraines did not come on overnight, and certainly a lifestyle approach can lead to a lifetime cure. The rewards of a headache-free existence make it worth any inconvenience at first to establish an appropriate lifestyle for preventing future migraine suffering.

13

Frequently Asked Questions

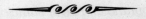

I n this chapter, we include questions we are asked over and over—as well as a few unusual questions people have asked us.

QUESTION: *My headaches don't fall into any of the usual patterns. I have a headache almost every day and a sick headache two or three times monthly. I have a severe unilateral throbbing headache associated with intense nausea, vomiting, and increased sensitivity to light and sound. What kind of headache is this, and what do I do about it?*

ANSWER: It sounds like you have more than one type of headache. The daily headaches are probably related to muscle contraction, which is discussed elsewhere in the book. The more infrequent unilateral headaches certainly sound like migraines.

Individuals who suffer from migraines are frequently more prone to other types of headaches such as daily muscle contraction headaches. Some forms of therapy are good for both types of headaches—such as tricyclic medications or aspirin, as well as techniques resulting in stress reduction, while other types of therapy, such as ergotamine or Sumatriptan, would be specific for migraine.

QUESTION: *I have suffered from migraines for approximately ten years. Some medications such as Cafergot and Sumatriptan have been somewhat helpful with the acute attacks. However, I still suffer from migraines two to three times monthly and miss at least one day a month from work because of these headaches.*

I have tried propranolol, Elavil, Pamelor, Prozac, and two or three other medications that I cannot recall. Moreover, I have tried limiting various items from my diet without success.

I have also tried biofeedback, acupuncture, and even other less mainstream forms of therapy without success. What do I do now?

ANSWER: The most important thing for you is not to give up, but to continue to educate yourself about your condition. Frequently, changes in diet, activity, or a new medication overlooked previously can have a dramatic effect on the course and control of migraine therapy. Moreover, new therapies are constantly being added to our anti-migrainous arsenal. As with any chronic medical condition, a positive attitude and vigilance usually pay off in one way or another.

QUESTION: *I have had migraines since childhood. My headaches have been quite severe and have interfered with work as well as my life in general.*

My mother has headaches similar to mine, as does my only sister. My headaches have been such a nuisance in my life that I would consider not having children because of my fear of passing on this torment to a child.

What is the risk of my child having migraine?

ANSWER: Unfortunately, there is no uniform genetic marker or specific body fluid test to identify all migraineurs. The inheritance pattern of migraine is far from clear. It is known that individuals with identical genetic makeup (identical or monozygotic twins) are more likely to both suffer from migraines than is the case with genetically dissimilar twins (nonidentical or dizygotic). Therefore a complex mode of inheritance must be considered. However, some studies have suggested that the risk of a child of a migraineur being afflicted with migraine is 45 percent while this number would increase to 70 percent if both patients have migraine.

QUESTION: *I have been told that I have classic migraine. My aura consists of wavy lines and other peculiar visual changes. If I take subcutaneous Sumatriptan early in the aura, will this affect the course of the aura and/or headache?*

ANSWER: This issue was recently addressed in an article in *Neurology* and consisted of a controlled study performed by doctors in England, Germany, Norway, and Denmark. This study did not find any significant alteration in nature or duration of the migraine or subsequent headache if 6 mg of Sumatriptan was injected subcutaneously during an aura (*Neurology 44*, 1994, pp. 1487–1592).

QUESTION: *My doctor tells me that because my headaches are invariably on the same side, it's very possible that I have a brain tumor or another serious abnormality on the side of my headaches. He tells me that migraine never affects just one side. What should I do?*

ANSWER: Past generations of neurologists have used the invariable laterality sign as an indication of a structural process, that is, tumor, abnormal blood vessel, causing the patient's headaches. Studies have indicated approximately 20 percent of patients' with super migraines have their headaches always on the same side. If you have never had an MRI scan,I would recommend this at some point.

QUESTION: *I have suffered migraines for most of my adult life. During my recent pregnancy, my migraines almost completely stopped. After delivery, however, my headaches are back with a vengeance. Imitrex has been helpful in the past for me; however, I am breast-feeding now. Is it safe to take Imitrex?*

ANSWER: It is known that Imitrex has been identified in the breast milk of animals. We have no information, unfortunately, about this in humans. Until evidence of Imitrex's safety in nursing women, this medication should probably be avoided.

QUESTION: *I'm a 34-year-old woman who suffers from migraine attacks, as well as from bulimia. Is there a connection?*

ANSWER: A recent publication has suggested there may be a link between the two illnesses. Of the thirty-four migraine patients surveyed in an eating disorder clinic, 88 percent admitted dieting, 59 percent admitted to food binging, and 26 percent reported having induced vomiting at some point in their life.

The migraineurs also scored high on half of the Eating Disorder Inventory Questionnaire, particularly with regard to body dissatisfaction, perfectionism, interpersonal distrust, and ineffectiveness. The authors conclude that a possible biochemical disorder may be involved. (For more information on causes of migraines, read chapter 2.)

QUESTION: *I know my headaches are related to food allergies. Really, I'm allergic to everything. My doctor is treating me with medications and other stuff, which I know will never work. I'm having severe headaches and missing work several times a month. What should I do?*

ANSWER: As we've discussed elsewhere in this book, the issue of food allergy-related migraine is very complex and controversial. We do feel that food allergy can play a role in migraine, but on a fairly infrequent basis.

The best approach for a migraine syndrome is to keep an open mind and be thorough with regard to exploring all possible factors that might be contributing to the frequency and severity of your headaches. If you are convinced that a particular treatment is not going to help you, then you will probably be right because of your negative attitude. Having a positive attitude about a new treatment is very important.

QUESTION: *My cat has frequent spells in which she vomits, becomes listless or irritable, and hides under the bed. These spells can last from twelve to twenty-four hours. Could my cat have migraine?*

ANSWER: This is certainly an interesting question. We are not aware of migraines existing in any type of animal, although animals do share other illnesses with humans. As we have described previously, the diagnosis of migraine is based primarily on history, and of course that is not available in this case, since the cat can't provide a detailed (or any!) history.

It is true that many mammals often are afflicted with neurologic disease similar to those of humans, including stroke and seizures. However, we have performed a literature search of the National Library of Medicine and been unable to find any reference to migraine in animals.

QUESTION: *I have both migraine and epilepsy and am on several different medications to treat the two conditions. Is there any way that my medication regimen can be simplified so that I don't have to take five medications, including some that might be good for my migraine but could make my seizures worse?*

ANSWER: It is fairly well accepted that some association exists between migraine and epilepsy. This recognition has important implications for physicians treating patients with either diagnosis. On one hand, a patient with epilepsy should be questioned extensively about possibly concurrent headaches while on the other hand the migraine patient should be questioned about possible symptoms of epilepsy.

A recent powerful study conducted by Ottman and Lipton has confirmed a close connection between epilepsy and migraines, but did not explain the nature of the association. There does not appear to be any relationship between the type of seizures, their cause, the patient's age at first seizure, or even family history of seizures and migraines.

As we mentioned previously, valproic acid (Depakote) appears to be helpful for both conditions. This medication is not good for all types of seizures but certainly is an effective tool in the management of many cases of epilepsy.

Moreover, it seems to decrease the frequency and severity of migraine attacks. Certainly a patient with migraines should avoid tricyclic medications as they could potentially make your seizures worse.

QUESTION: *I have heard about a new test for diagnosing migraine called transcranial doppler. Should I have this test done?*

ANSWER: Probably not. Transcranial doppler (TCD) is a method to study the arterial blood supply of the brain. By sending pulses of sound waves into the skull from various sites, the echo can be analyzed to provide some information about the speed of blood flow.

At least one study has suggested that the blood flow velocities in migraineurs is markedly increased. While this is certainly interesting, its diagnostic implications at this point are unresolved. Performing a TCD in a suspected migraine patient is, at this point, still experimental.

QUESTION: *Can the visual changes which occur in patients with migraine headache disorder be permanent?*

ANSWER: While permanent visual changes are very infrequent, it is true that persistent visual phenomena occur in rare individuals who suffer from migraine headache disorder. This problem can last from weeks to months and even up to years. As was recently reported in the April 1995 *Neurology Journal* (the premiere journal for neurology specialists), these phenomena occur in select and unfortunate individuals.

Oftentimes, people will seek the attention of an ophthalmologist (eye doctor) prior to realizing that these are indeed related to their migraine headache syndrome. If the visual disturbance persists, medical attention should be sought.

QUESTION: *When should I be concerned about my headache?*

ANSWER: Headaches are a sign of an underlying illness process and should always merit your attention. However, as neurologists, we feel that headaches are of concern primarily if they meet certain criteria, which include the following:

- The worst headache ever
- A sudden thunderclap or immediate onset of headache, which becomes intractable
- Headache symptoms that first occur after the age of 45
- Headaches associated with progressive severity
- Headaches associated with neurologic signs or symptoms, which would include numbness, weakness, tingling, burning, stumbling, falling, loss of balance or coordination, and severe visual changes
- Headaches that worsen with cough, sneeze, or straining with a bowel movement
- Any headache that concerns you, particularly if it follows an atypical course or persists for more than 24–36 hours

QUESTION: *My doctor, who has worked with me for some time, has suggested a headache center for my problem with frequent headaches. Do these clinics help?*

ANSWER: Patients are often referred to us for an inpatient evaluation. That means, we decide whether or not to admit patients to the hospital for management of their severe headache disorder. While a comprehensive team approach with the specialist, psychologist, social worker, exercise physiologist, and physical therapist is often helpful, we use inpatient therapy and hospital admission only as a last resort.

Frequently, a careful medical history will provide valuable clues for treating and resolving your severe headache syndrome. Also, it is important that you keep an accurate headache diary, an example of which can be found in the Appendix.

QUESTION: *How long after I change my diet and follow a specific headache diet should I see results?*

ANSWER: This is difficult to determine. As noted elsewhere in this book, some migraine sufferers will only have a headache every three to six months, and others will have a headache even less frequently.

We feel that a headache elimination diet of triggers will take anywhere from 6–12 weeks before one could even begin to assess its true efficacy. However, in certain individuals, a headache diet takes even longer to be completely effective, and it is more a matter of degree than an all-or-none phenomenon.

If you are getting some benefit with your diet, and there is any reduction in severity, intensity, or frequency of your headaches, we urge that you "stick with it."

QUESTION: *I have been reading in some magazines that one of the treatments for migraine is to replace magnesium. Can I* *give myself a magnesium injection, and how do I go about doing this?*

ANSWER: While you are correct in your assumption that magnesium may place a role in the production and ultimately termination of migraine headache pain, we strongly urge our patients to avoid self-medication until we know exactly whether or not their magnesium level is low.

We don't allow our patients to provide magnesium injections. Instead, these injections must be provided by a physician. Often, when a low magnesium level has been detected, we will allow our patients to take a multivitamin supplement with magnesium as part of the supplement.

If there is any question as to whether or not you have a low magnesium level, your physician certainly can draw a blood test to assess this.

QUESTION: *I have heard that there are medicines that can be taken as a nasal spray to terminate migraine headaches. Can you tell me what these are, and how do they act?*

ANSWER: There are a few intranasal medication treatments, the most common being Stadol nasal spray (butorphanol). This acts as a narcotic medication to manage the headache pain, which can often be successful in terminating a migraine headache.

In addition, this is often successful in combination with other medication, particularly as a secondary medication (such as after an Imitrex injection). Additional medications that are useful in the nasal form are dihydroergotamine nasal spray. (This medication is not yet available in the U.S. but is used widely with promising results in other countries.)

Other preparations may soon be available for specific termination of migraine headache pain. Please consult your physician as to the exact dosage for your height and weight and medical history.

QUESTION: *If I have a headache disorder, does that mean that I need to have a picture of my brain (CAT scan or other study)?*

ANSWER: No. Most people who have common migraine headache disorders rarely need to undergo special imaging studies (CAT scan, x-rays, magnetic scans of the brain or neck).

Unless your headache involves other signs or symp–toms such as numbness, incoordination, clumsiness, tingling, burning, weakness, or dizziness, you most likely can be followed clinically. Nevertheless, this is something you should discuss with your physician, particularly after reviewing a complete medical history.

QUESTION: *Can poor sleeping habits play some role in my frequent recurrent headaches?*

ANSWER: Absolutely. One of the issues which we discuss in our chapter on lifestyle changes is controlling your sleep cycle, and we have provided multiple clues as to how to do this.

We feel that the expression "If only I could get a good night's sleep, I know I would feel better" is certainly not an old wives' tale. We feel that good sleep is absolutely mandatory to effect a positive change in patients who suffer from migraine headaches. We often prescribe sleep medications, such as Ambien, to help patients adjust their sleep cycle and hopefully return their sleep pattern to normal.

QUESTION: *My dentist told me I have TMJ. Can this be playing any role in my headaches?*

ANSWER: Definitely. In addition, many people do not know that they are grinding their teeth (bruxism) during sleep. Oftentimes, a simple bite block or mouthpiece, which can be fitted for individual patients and worn at nighttime, can prevent the jaw grinding, thereby reducing the jaw pain the TMJ pain, and subsequently the risk of daily headaches.

The mechanism of action of jaw joint pain producing headaches is one that is related to the muscle contraction theory of headache. When the muscles over the jaw joints go into spasm, they trigger other muscles to tighten up, causing contraction of muscles along the base of the skull, the back of the neck, and into the shoulders.

This then produces triggers, waste toxins, and waste products, and leads to severe head and neck pain. This can be a vicious cycle and certainly needs to be addressed. A competent dentist and maxillofacial surgeon (dental specialist in jaw alignment) can often alleviate this problem without the use of medications, and can often break the headache cycle promptly.

QUESTION: *My husband smokes, and I tell him to stop it. I always seem to do worse when he smokes and I wonder if his smoking can be playing any role in my headaches.*

ANSWER: Yes. Women are more susceptible to cigarette smoke as a trigger than men, and in addition, are more susceptible to chemicals, odors, and perfumes that may act as triggers for their severe headache and migraine pain.

Additional triggers and precipitating factors for migraine that are more common in women than in men include the following: weather changes, missed meals, perfume, cigarette smoke, sunlight, stress, and sleeping too little. Triggers that are more common in men than in women include headaches associated with exercise and with sexual activity.

QUESTION: *How can I identify what is causing my headache?*

ANSWER: This is a complex question that is discussed in several chapters of this book. However, briefly, we offer the following advice:

- Keep a headache diary.
- Ask friends and family members to comment regarding moods, behaviors, and activities that occur immediately before or during headache attacks.
- Chart cycles in your headache, including their relationship to the weekdays vs. weekends, the menstrual cycle (if you are a woman), pay day, and so on. Monitor your diet, activity, and sleep cycle. Then discuss all the above information with your physician, to see if together you can find your headache triggers and determine an effective treatment.

QUESTION: *I have my headaches at the time of my menstrual cycle. Is there anything in particular that is helpful for this?*

ANSWER: Yes. As we have discussed elsewhere in this book, many women will suffer what is called catamenial migraine. There is actually very specific treatment for certain individuals who have this, which includes the following:

Anti-inflammatory medications

Ergotamine preparations

Dihydroergotamine

Methergine

Methysergide

Standard preventative medicines such as tricyclic medications (Elavil, Pamelor), calcium channel blockers (verapamil, Calan, etc.), beta-blockers (Inderal, Tenormin, Lopressor).

Parlodel is often very effective for catamenial migraine, although this medicine is much more commonly used in patients with Parkinson's disease.

In addition, we have had very good success with Diamox, a type of water pill, which can reduce the swelling and the bloating of menses, as well as prevent a migraine headache.

If these medications are not effective, some authorities will recommend using such strong medicines such as steroid medications, as well as tranquilizers. We try to avoid these in our practice.

QUESTION: *Who treats migraine headaches?*

ANSWER: Oftentimes, general practitioners and family physicians will attempt to initiate the treatment and management of headache pain. However, if the pain syndrome requires medications, physician visits, and is involved with any type of lifestyle change or medical disability, the specialist who treats headache disorders (migraine and non-migraine headaches) is a neurologist.

Neurologists are specialists who deal with the central and peripheral nervous system, that is, the brain, the spinal cord, the nerve roots, the nerve twigs, and the muscles that are supplied by these.

The Academy of Neurology, an excellent resource, as well as other agencies helpful in answering questions regarding headache disorders, are listed in the Appendix.

QUESTION: *I tend to have more migraines when I travel. Why is this?*

ANSWER: There are many reasons for this. When we travel, we all tend to change our routine activities and get out of our normal lifestyle pattern. We seem to have changes in our appetite, our eating behaviors, and the foods we eat.

In addition, our sleep cycle is often changed or deranged entirely. Our exercise activity is quite different than in our home and natural environment. Often when we travel, we are exposed to changes in altitude and climates, as well as temperature changes.

Another point to keep in mind is that to arrive at a destination, we often travel by car, train, or airplane, and are exposed to various motions, all of which can act as migraine triggers. It is rarely one isolated aspect of the travel that produces these triggers, so identifying carefully all aspects that seem to play a role can often lead to alleviating this phenomenon.

QUESTION: *Can yeast infections cause migraines?*

ANSWER: Any stress to the body can act as a trigger for migraine pain. Patients who have upper respiratory infections or influenza, women who are menstruating, and individuals under psycho-social stressors are all more susceptible to migraine syndrome.

One popularly held theory is that this yeast infection is actually a connection to the immune system, acting to trigger our immune response and start this cascade effect, which we discuss under "Theories of Migraine." Another concept is that the yeast connection acts as a variant of an allergic reaction where the body initiates an allergic response at some level to trigger headache disorders. While yeast infections may indeed be a trigger in certain individuals, the jury is still out as to what the complete role of yeast infections in migraine pain disorders truly is.

QUESTION: *My doctor has recommended that I get a shot to treat my headache pain. Do you know what he is talking about, and how would this work?*

ANSWER: We are not exactly sure which type of shot your physician is recommending. As a general overview, perhaps the following will be helpful:

We use different types of injections for managing not only migraines but also daily headache pain syndromes. Of course, this is not our first choice of therapy.

Some injections are simply narcotic injections for the pain management. Narcotics comes from the Greek word "narcos," which means "to sleep," and the narcotic injection will simply put the pain to sleep for a short period of time. We prefer not to use these, as these can be habit-forming and addicting. They are often effective, but frequently will have significant side effects.

Additional injections include medicines given through the vein, such as intravenous magnesium or intravenous medicines to prevent nausea and to produce sleep. These have been discussed elsewhere in this book.

Other injections provide a neuro-blockade (blockage of the pain messengers and the pain information transmission from the brain throughout the rest of the body). These often include medications that produce anesthesia (such as xylocaine or lidocaine, which most patients receive as they get a dental procedure), and are fairly well tolerated.

Neuro-blockade injections frequently produce only a period of anesthesia or numbness. The numbing medication may often be given with a second injection, that being a steroid-type medication, which can provide long-acting anti-inflammatory effect, preventing inflammation in the muscles, ligaments, tendons, and joints that often are secondary phenomena from muscle spasm and muscle contractions.

These injections are often given at the base of the skull, as well as in the mid-portion of the back of the neck. The Academy of Anesthesiology often recommends that these be administered as a series of three shots, but we suggest that our patients have a trial of an initial injection, and if this works, then a second and third injection may be helpful.

Finally, local trigger injections, often with just local anesthetic agents such as xylocaine or lidocaine or marcaine, are helpful to alleviate pain at an isolated trigger point. All of these therapies are best discussed with your physician and indeed even better discussed with a specialist who performs these pain injections, such as an individual who has completed a fellowship in pain management.

QUESTION: *I have frequent sick headaches. My doctor does not seem to take them seriously and often states: "Well, here's a different medication." What can I do to convince my doctor that these are disabling, and how do I go about getting rid of my headaches?*

ANSWER: This is a complex question, as we have discussed elsewhere in this book. However, briefly, in the doctor/patient relationship, you bring the most important aspect—the patient. It is important that you provide accurate and concise information regarding your symptom complex.

Nevertheless, if you cannot convince your physician to appreciate the severity of your illness, or if you do not feel that you and your physician are communicating effectively, as we have stated early in chapter 8 on "Choosing the Right Doctor," it is probably time to find a new or additional physician, one who has particular interest or expertise in treating patients who suffer from headache disorders.

Also, it would be helpful to present your new doctor with a comprehensive headache diary, one that demonstrates how different aspects of your life and lifestyle are affected by your headaches. This would include information regarding diet, exercise, activity, sleep cycle, work cycle, days missed from work, and activities that had to be changed or canceled because of your headache pain. This often is effective in convincing your physician that this is indeed "a serious problem."

QUESTION: *I have suffered from migraines, and now my 9-year-old son has apparently developed a migraine headache disorder. Are there different medicines for him than there are for me?*

ANSWER: Actually, the medication management for migraine in young children in somewhat different than it is for adults. While many physicians like to use Inderal, a relatively safe and effective medication for the prevention of migraine, it does indeed have some side effects. Also, this is a medication that should be avoided in children with asthma.

Nevertheless, oftentimes behavior modification, removal of triggers, and change in lifestyle patterns can be effective in alleviating the migraine disorder in children, and this can alleviate the need for medication management. In addition, it is important to recognize that migraines in children may be experienced as abdominal discomfort, malaise, fatigue, and a general sense of being unwell, and may not present with the complete spectrum of a migraine disorder that adults seem to experience.

This should be discussed with your pediatrician, and possibly a neurologist or pediatric neurologist would be helpful in evaluating your son's condition.

QUESTION: *My eye doctor told me that my vision changes could be a migraine attack. How could this be and what do I do for it?*

ANSWER: Your eye doctor may be right. Ophthalmic migraines are not uncommon, although permanent effects from ophthalmic migraines are quite rare. The diagnosis for ophthalmic/retinal migraine includes reversible single eye blindness or vision changes lasting less than 60 minutes, with the patient able to clearly identify a visual disturbance and draw the visual disturbance.

The headache will often follow the visual symptoms within 60 minutes, but may indeed precede the visual disturbance. There is an entirely normal eye examination away from the attack. This may be due to spasm or reduction in the blood flow to the retinal artery (the artery that supplies blood and oxygen to the eye), and there may be swelling of the artery wall. Standard anti-migraine therapy such as beta-blockers, calcium channel blockers, and aspirin therapy are often quite helpful. This condition should be discussed with your physician.

Appendix 1:
Activities for Daily Living

———◦◦◦———

This section includes basic and helpful advice for migraineurs, as well as people who suffer from muscle contraction headaches.

The following section will discuss proper body mechanics for your daily activities. In some cases, the mechanical stresses (load) to the spine for various positions has been included. This will give you an understanding of the importance of adequate strength, flexibility, and proper alignment in order to: (1) reduce load, (2) improve function, (3) alleviate pain and discomfort, and (4) prevent further injury.

The standard mechanical stress load to the spine is 100 percent when standing with correct posture.

Walking Posture

As you begin to walk, consciously pull your head, neck, and shoulders back. Heel should strike first while pushing off with the toes of the back foot. As you step forward, lift trunk tall and pull abdominals in.

This may feel strange at first, but remember you are not used to walking or moving with correct alignment. Eventually this will feel natural.

Prolonged Standing Technique

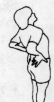

While standing for prolonged periods of time, stagger feet shoulder width apart and shift weight from one leg to the other. To alleviate pressure on the lower back while ironing or doing dishes, stand close to the ironing board or sink with one leg elevated 2–4 inches off the floor. Avoid leaning forward from the pelvis, back, or shoulders.

NOTE: Keep a soft knee, abdominals in, shoulders back, and raised sternum (breast bone). Keep your head and neck back.

Frequent One-Minute Breaks

The one-minute break is designed to enable you to change position frequently. Take time to get up and move around. Perform a few of the exercises you have learned. Use the corner stretch to help you stretch the chest and straighten your posture. Walk around your desk or office. Go to the bathroom.

Do anything that gets you moving.

Using the Telephone

When talking on the telephone, keep your head level, with shoulders and neck back.

Try not to hold the telephone with your shoulder elevated and head tilted to the side. This holds stress and tension in the upper back and neck.

Sleeping

Improper sleeping posture increases the mechanical stress on
the spine. The tightness in the
soft tissues of the pelvis and legs,
coupled with poor hip alignment,
can be a source of discomfort
along the whole spine. This can
lead to neck spasm. The following rules will aid in supporting
the spine and pelvis as well as
reducing the mechanical stress to
the spine.

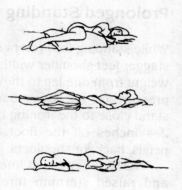

1. Sleep on a firm mattress to reduce tension caused by excessive curvature.
   - If you sleep on your side: place a pillow in between your knees. This will reduce the mechanical stress to 75 percent.
   - If you sleep on your back: place a pillow under your knees. This will reduce the mechanical stress to 5 percent. With legs extended, stress increases to 150 percent.
   - If you sleep on your abdomen: place a pillow under-neath your hips.

Ideal Sitting and Driving Posture

Sitting causes the greatest increase in spine
pressure (up to 275 percent); therefore, proper

sitting posture is essential in order to reduce chronic back pain. Knees should be slightly higher than the hips, and your back should be firmly supported by the back of the chair or seat. The chair back should ideally be on an incline and have arm rests.

Keep head and neck retracted and abdominals in. While driving, keep both hands on the steering wheel, in the 10 and 2 o'clock positions, for support. Be certain that you are close enough to the foot pedals so that you do not have to reach for them.

Note: Sit in correct posture. Adjust all mirrors to accommodate this posture. The mirrors will act as a reminder to correct your position when your posture fails. Also, place a rolled towel in the natural curve of your lower back to add support and to remind you to remain in correct posture.

Mechanical Stress to the Low Back:
Sitting with Proper Posture: 140 percent
Sitting with Improper Posture: up to 275 percent

Getting Out of Bed or Off the Couch

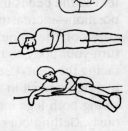

Using proper mechanics to get out of bed will reduce unnecessary tension on the spine. Before getting out of bed, bring knees to chest and grasp legs under knees. Pull into chest and raise shoulders to meet knees. Hold 10–30 seconds, release, then repeat. This will help you get ready to move. Roll onto your side and use your free arm to help push your torso up while you simultaneously swing your feet and legs off the bed or couch. This will leave you in a seated position.

Standing and Sitting

Using the proper technique to stand
and/or sit will strengthen the legs
and reduce discomfort and stress on
the vertebrae.

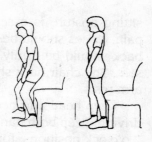

　　To stand: Move to the edge of the
chair. Place feet shoulder-width apart
with one foot slightly in front of the other (back foot should be
placed slightly under chair). Lean forward from the hips. Lift
body with your legs. Stand erect and in good posture.

　　To sit: Stand tall with shoulder blades squeezing together.
Back calf against the chair. Feet should be shoulder-width
apart with one foot slightly in front of the other foot. Pull abdominals in, push hips back, and bend knees. Using the legs,
ease back into the chair.

Getting In and Out of a Car or Confined Space

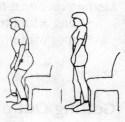

Always get in and out of a car without
twisting or separating the legs. This
leaves the pelvis in an unsupported
position—increasing the mechanical
stress on the spine. To get into a car,
turn your body so that your back is
facing the seat. Use proper sitting
technique to sit in the car seat, then
swing both legs into the car simultaneously. Getting out of the car is the exact
opposite. Begin by moving both legs out of the car
(using a full body turn). Place one foot in front of
the other, lean forward from the hips, and stand
erect. Keep shoulders back and chest elevated.

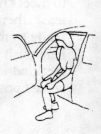

Half Kneeling

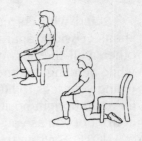

Move to the edge of your chair. Place one foot in front of the other with back leg under chair. With back flat and abs in tight, lean forward from the hips while pressing through the heel on your front leg, lift up and back onto the chair. This technique is great for getting clothes out of the dryer, getting things out of low cabinets, and so on.

Getting Off the Floor

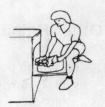

Half kneeling is a precursor to getting off the floor.

Roll onto all fours. Pull abdominal muscles in tight, walk hands back toward knees, and move into a kneeling position using your bent leg for support. You can now get into a chair or stand straight up using the half-kneeling technique.

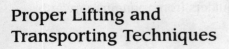

Proper Lifting and Transporting Techniques

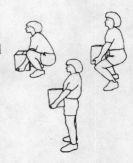

Lifting in any position will increase the mechanical load on the spine. The mechanical advantage to lifting with proper technique is to reduce the compressive forces on the spine and increase the stability of the spine during lifting and transport.

Stand with correct posture (see wall stance), place feet shoulder-width apart with one foot slightly in front of the other. Pull the abs in tight and lean forward from the hips while bending the knees (squatting down). Pick up the object (using your legs to lift), tighten abs, and exhale as you slowly lift to an upright position. Keep object close to your body and in front of you as you transport item to its new location.

NOTE: Shifting the weight load to one side increases disc pressure and muscle activity on the opposite side.

Lift slowly and in a controlled manner; disc pressure increases with faster lifts and heavier loads.

Other Helpful Hints

- Lighten pocketbook and switch shoulders frequently. This will keep you from leaning and/or favoring one side.

- Avoid wearing high heels (higher than one inch above the sole of the shoe). These tend to tilt the pelvis forward and increase the curvature in the low back.

- Obesity greatly increases both the direct and indirect compressive loads on the spine by shifting center of gravity and increasing the curvature of the spine. Weight loss could reduce your pain.

- Stand with your arms behind your back. This will help you to keep your shoulders from rounding forward.

Appendix 2:
Neck Knowledge
and Neck Exercises

Neck pain can result from acute injuries or trauma (falls, whiplash) or from improper body mechanics or improper position (poor sleeping posture, poor spinal alignment). And neck pain can contribute to headache pain.

Whatever the basis for your neck pain, it can typically be reduced with a flexibility, strengthening, and proper spinal alignment exercise program. By increasing the strength of the supporting structures of the spine (muscles, tendons, ligaments, discs, vertebrae), the mechanical loads and stressors are taken off the head and neck, thereby possibly resulting in reduced pain. Exercise activity can also produce proper spinal alignment of the neck, which can lead to marked reduction in neck pain and prevention of future injury. A strong neck is a healthy neck, and with this, one can resist the forces of injury.

Week One

1. *Shoulder Shrugs* (for flexibility and strength)

    Movement: With arms relaxed at your side, lift shoulder to ear and circle back and down. Repeat 10 times. Hint: Squeeze shoulder blades together on the rotation backward. At no time should shoulder rotate forward.

2. *Flexion and Extension*

    Movement: Move chin to chest and push shoulder down. As you elevate chin to ceiling, shrug shoulders and hold for 1–2 seconds to enhance the stretch in extended position, push chin up. Repeat 10 times in each direction.

    Note: This can also be used as a stretch. Hold each position for 10–20 seconds.

3. *Lateral Flexion*

    Movement: Shoulders should be relaxed and down. Lift right ear to ceiling and left ear to shoulder. Hold for 1–2 seconds, then move back to center. Repeat on other side.

    Note: This can also be used as a stretch. Hold each position for 10–20 seconds.

4. *Neck Rotation*

    Movement: Rotate chin and ear to side, hold 1–2 seconds, then look down at shoulder. Move back to center. Rotate in the opposite direction.

    Note: This can also be used as a stretch. Hold each position for 10–20 seconds.

5. *Neck Retraction*

Movement: Squeeze shoulder blades together. Pull head straight back keeping jaw
and eyes level. Hold for 5–10 seconds and
relax. Repeat 10 times. Try to focus on
proper posture during retraction.
    Hint: Do not drop or lift chin.

6. *Chest and Shoulder Stretch*

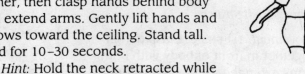

Movement: Squeeze shoulder blades together, then clasp hands behind body
and extend arms. Gently lift hands and
elbows toward the ceiling. Stand tall.
Hold for 10–30 seconds.
    Hint: Hold the neck retracted while
squeezing shoulder blades together.
    Modification: This can also be done by placing hands
on a doorway and passing torso through entrance.

Week Two

7. *Shoulder Retraction*

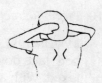

Movement: With fingers touching the
ears and elbows up, pinch shoulder
blades together (as you do this, your elbows will move back). Hold for 5 seconds and release shoulder blades. Do
not pull or push on the neck.
    Hint: Hold the neck retracted (see exercise 5) while
squeezing shoulder blades together.
    Modification: If it is painful to have hands behind your
ears, then place hands on shoulders.

8. *Neck Stretch*

Movement: Lift right ear to ceiling. Grasp right arm above wrist (in front of body) and drop shoulders as you gently pull your right arm down. Hold for ten seconds. Repeat with same arm behind back. Repeat to the other side.

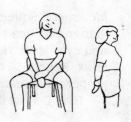

Hint: To enhance this stretch, rotate chin up and down.

9. *Upper Back Stretch*

Movement: 1st stage: Clasp hands together in front of body with both arms extended. Gently pull shoulder blades apart and drop chin to chest. Hold for 10–30 seconds.

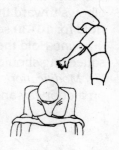

2nd stage: Sit in a chair, cross arms, and grab arm rests. Move your chin to your chest as you open shoulder blades.

10. *Prone Retraction*

Movement: Lie on the corner of a bed, face down, head and neck relaxed. With arms bent and elbows raised, squeeze shoulder blades together, raising elbows, and hold for 5 seconds. Build up to holding for 15 seconds. Repeat 5 times.

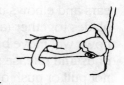

Hint: Place a pillow under your hips for support. Repeat exercise 9.

11. *Abdominal Crunches*

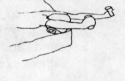

Movement: Lie on your beck
with knees bent and feet flat on
the floor. With hands at your
side, lift your head and shoulders off the floor, moving
hands either toward ankles or knees as you lift.

   Hint: Head should be in a rigid position (pretend
to have an apple between your chin and chest while
lifting).

   Note: It is normal for the neck muscles to become
fatigued.

12. *Arm Lift*

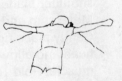

Movement: Lie on the corner of a bed
face down, with head and neck relaxed. Extend arms over your head
and raise arms toward the ceiling.
Hold for 2–5 seconds, increasing to
15 seconds over time. Repeat 5 times.

   Hint: Place a pillow under your hips for support.
Repeat exercise 6 and 9.

13. *Stabilization of Shoulder Girdle*

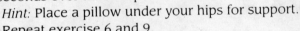

Movement: Lie on the corner of a
bed face down. Relax head and
neck. With arms extended out to
the side, squeeze shoulder blades
together and raise both arms toward the ceiling. Hold for
5–10 seconds. Build up to holding for 20 seconds.

   Note: This exercise will become easier over time. It
can be advanced by holding soup cans and then weights.
Reduce your hold time to 1–3 seconds.

   Hint: Place a pillow under your hips for support.
Repeat exercise 9.

14. *Upper Back and Neck Stretch*

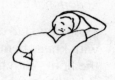

Movement: Tilt head to the side and gently grasp the side of your head (at ear) and allow gravity to stretch the muscles. Then place opposite hand behind back. Hold for 10–20 seconds.

   Note: Do not pull on head and neck!

15. *Shoulder Reach*

Movement: Lie on your back with arms extended toward the ceiling. Attempt to open your shoulder blades as you push arms straight up to the ceiling. Keep your back against the floor and elbows straight. Hold for 5 seconds and build up to 15 seconds.

   Repeat exercise 6.

16. *Shoulder Blade Lift*

Movement: Place left hand of left shoulder blade, elevating elbow. Move chin and nose to right shoulder. Gently place right hand on top of head and allow gravity to stretch the muscle. Hold 10–20 seconds, repeat to the other side.

   Note: Do not pull on head and neck.

17. *Upward Row*

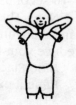

Movement: (1) Stand tall with shoulder blades squeezing together. Hold a towel with both hands in front of your body, palms facing toward the body. Leading with the elbows, lift both hands to the chin and hold; squeeze shoulder blades together in this position.

(2) Once this becomes familiar, add 1–5 pound weights, repeat 10–20 times.

Form Check: At the height of the exercise, elbows should be higher than the ears and wrists.

Repeat stretches 8 and 14.

Appendix 3:
Life Guide Adult
Daily Dietary Supplements

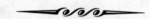

Vitamins

- Beta carotene—25,000 units each day with the main meal
- Vitamin E—400 units each day with the main meal
- Vitamin C—1,000 to 2,000 milligrams with morning meal
- Vitamin B Complex (B1, 50 milligrams; B2, 50 milligrams; B6, 100 milligrams; B12, 100 micrograms; niacinamide, 100 milligrams; folic acid, 100 micrograms) with morning meal

Minerals

- Magnesium—400 to 600 milligrams with morning meal (amino acid chelate)

- Copper—3 milligrams with morning meal (amino acid chelate)
- Manganese—30 to 40 milligrams with morning meal (amino acid chelate)
- Zinc—30 to 50 milligrams with morning meal (amino acid chelate)
- Potassium—50 to 100 milligrams with morning meal (amino acid chelate)
- Chromium picolinate—100 to 150 micrograms with morning meal
- Selenium—100 to 150 micrograms with morning meal (amino acid chelate)
- Boron—2 to 3 milligrams with morning meal
- Molybdenum—25 to 50 micrograms with morning meal (amino acid chelate)
- Vanadium—50 to 100 micrograms with morning meal (amino acid chelate)
- Silicon—1 milligram with morning meal (amino acid chelate). This is one health food vitamin supplement, available at health food stores and at the following address:

Appendix 4:
Headache Diary

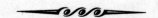

The opposite page shows an example of the headache diary we frequently ask patients to use. A completed diary is a diagnostic tool that helps us track the patient's symptoms. By examining when a headache began, its possible triggers, and the character and duration of pain, we can better identify the exact type of headache, which in turn makes our treatment more accurate and effective.

The large grid is self-explanatory. The smaller grids on the right help you track the frequency and severity of your headaches over a three-month period. This is done with a simple rating scale of 0 to 10, where 0 = no pain, and 10 = agony. For the calendar tracking to work, you need to enter a number on the calendar every day.

Headache Diary

NAME: _____   DATE: FROM _____ TO _____

Month _____

S	M	T	W	TH	F	S

Month _____

S	M	T	W	TH	F	S

Month _____

S	M	T	W	TH	F	S

DATE/ TIME:	HEADACHE DURATION – DID IT RETURN?	LOCATION OF HEADACHE PAIN:	CHARACTER OF PAIN Examples: throbbing, Estabbing, dull, sharp	HEADACHE TRIGGER:	I GOT BETTER WITH:

Appendix 5:
Headache Questionnaire

1. At what age did your headaches first begin?

2. What was the initial frequency of your headaches?

3. Is this frequency increasing, decreasing, or staying the same?

4. Do you experience more than one type of headache?

5. Do you have any triggers:
   a. Food
   b. Environmental (i.e., weather, heat, odors.)
   c. Stress
   d. Activities
   e. In relation to menstrual cycle
   f. Other:

6. Have you found an effective treatment?

7. If the answer to #6 was yes, what is that treatment:

8. Have you had any diagnostic testing thus far?
   a. X-rays
   b. CT brain
   c. MRI brain
   d. EEG
   e. Laboratory tests
   f. Other:

9. Have you gone more than 3 months at a time without any headaches?

10. Have you tried any nonmedical treatments for your migraine:
    a. Herbal medicines
    b. Stress management techniques
    c. Exercise
    d. Yoga/meditation
    e. Breathing techniques
    f. Other:

11. Is there any relationship between work activities and your headaches (eg. sitting, manual labor, etc.)?

12. If the answer to #11 was yes, what is the relationship?

13. Do you have a good sleep cycle?

14. If the answer to #12 is no, do you have trouble:
    a. Falling asleep
    b. Maintaining sleep
    c. Awakening too early

15. Have you ever had a problem with habit-forming medications?

16. How long was the longest headache you've experienced?

17. How short was the shortest headache you've experienced?

18. Do you have any unusual components to your headache:
    a. Vision changes
    b. Nausea
    c. Disorientation
    d. Weakness/numbness
    e. Other:

19. Are you concerned that your headaches represent a "brain tumor"?

List of Medicines

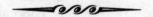

Medicines and drugs mentioned in the book are listed here alphabetically by their brand names and, in some cases, by their generic names, e.g., *Acetaminophen, Propranol, Quinine Sulphate* The medicines marked with asterik are not available in India under the same name at this point of time. To facilitate their identification, their generic composition is given.

Acetaminophen
ADALT (Adalt)
ADAPIN (Doxin, Doxetar,
   Spectra) *Doxepin*
ALEVE (Artagen, Movibon,
   Napryn, Naprosyn)
   Naproxen Sodium
AMBIEN* *Zolpidem Tartrate*
Aspirin

BELLERGAL-S* *Belladona*
   Alkaloids +Phenobarbital
Butalbital

CAFERGOT(Cafergot)
CALAN SR(Calaptin,
   Vasopten)*Verapamil HCl*
Captopril
Carbamazepine
CARDIZEM(Diltine, Angizem,
   Dicard, Channel)
   Diltiazem HCl
Cimetidine
Clonidine
Codeine
COMPAZINE (Stemetil,
   Emidoxyn) *Prochlorperazine*
Cyproheptadine

DARVOCET(Darvocet)

DARVON* *Propoxyphene HCl*
DAYPRO* *Oxaproxin*
DEMEROL* *Meperidine HCl*
DEPAKENE & DEPAKOTE
   (Valparin, Epilex,
   Encorate, Epival) *Valproic*
   Acid
Desipramine
DESYREL(Tazodac,
   Trazodep, Trazalon,
   Depryl-25) *Trazodone*
Dextromethorphan
DHE (Dhe)
DIAMOX(Diamox, Synomox,
   Opener)*Acetazolamide*
Dichloralphenazone
Diclofenac Sodium
Dihydroergotamine
DILANTIN(Dilantin)

ELAVIL(Amitone, Tridep,
   Eliwel, Latilin)*Amitriptyline*
ENDEP(Amitone, Tridep,
   Eliwel, Latilin)*Amitriptyline*
ERGOSTAT(In combination:
   Dhe, Ergophen, Migranil)
   Ergotamine
Ergotamine

ESGIC PLUS*Acetaminophen + Caffeine + Butalbital

FIORECET*Acetaminophen + Caffeine + Butalbital

FLORINAL 3*Aspirin + Caffeine + Butalbital + Codeine Phosphate

IMITREX(Imitrex)
INDERAL(Inderal)
INDOCIN(Articid, Idicin, Indocap)Indomethacin
Isometheptene Mucate
ISOPTIN(Isoptin)

Ketorolac

LIDOCAINE(Lidocaine)
LOPRESSOR(Lopressor)
LORCET*Hydrocodone Bitartrate+Acetaminophen

METHERGINE*Methylergonovine Maleate
Metoclopramide
MIDRIN*Isometheptene Mucate+Dichloralphenazone +Acetaminophen
MOTRIN(Brufen, Embru, Emflam)Ibuprofen

Naloxone or Natrexone
NAPROSYN*Naproxen
Naproxen Sodium
NARDIL*Phenelzine Sulfate
Nimodipine
Nitroglycerine
NORPRAMIN(Norpramin)

PAMELOR(Nortin, Primox, Sensival)Nortriptyline
PARLODEL(B-Crip, Brom, N-Crip, Scriptin) Bromocriptine Mesylate
PERCOCET*Oxycodone HCl +Acetaminophen
Percutaneous Estradiol Gel
PERIACTIN(Periactin)

Phenacetin
PHENERGAN(Phenergan)
Phenobarbital
Phenytoin
PROCARDIA(Adalt, Aginal, Calat, Depin) Nifedipine
Propranol
PROZAC(Fludac, Fluex, Flufran, Flunil) Fluoxetine

QUINAM(P-Falci, Qinarsol, Quininga, Rez-Q) Quinine Sulphate
Quinine Sulphate

REGLAN(Reglan)

SANSERT*Methysergide
SINEQUAN(Doxetor, Doxin, Spectra) Doxepin
Sumpatriptan

TEGRETOL(Tegretol)
TENORMIN(Tenormin)
Theophylline
THORAZINE(Emetil, Megatil, Sunprazin)Chlorpromazine
TIGAN*Trimethobenzamide HCI
TORADOL(Cadolac, Kelac, Ketanov, Ketro)Ketorolac
TYLENOL(Crocin, Algina, Atamol, Bepamol) Acetaminophen

Verapamil
VICODIN*Hydrocodone Bitartrate+Acetaminophen
VIVACTIL*Protriptyline
VOLTAREN (Diclomol, Voveran, Diclomove) Diclofenac Sodium

WIGRAINE (Migranil) Ergotamine Tartrate + Caffeine

Xylocaine

Glossary

abnormal blood vessels. An abnormal connection between arteries and veins or an abnormal artery with an out-pouching, leading to a weakened vessel and possible hemorrhage.

acupuncture. An Eastern style of therapy which uses special treatments of pressure and trigger points to release the body's own pain chemicals.

adrenaline. The body's stress chemical, which plays a role in our "fight or flight" natural instinct.

angiography. The study of a blood vessel from inside the artery; often a cousin to cardiac catheterizations, which look at the heart. Carotid and cerebral angiography look at the arteries of the neck and arteries of the brain, respectively.

antidepressants. Medications to reduce or relieve depression.

anti-emetics. Medicines that work to prevent or reduce nausea and vomiting.

aura. The premonition and sensation that a migraine headache will be following.

beta-blockers. A class of medicine that is used in migraine headache management. This is also used for blood pressure control and other illnesses.

breathing techniques. A special type of breathing pattern used to modulate pain and modulate and adjust the nervous system.

calcium channel blockers. A class of medicine used in migraine headache management, high blood pressure, and heart disease.

CAT scan. Computerized axial tomography scan, often used as a screening study to rule out hemorrhage in the brain and rule out brain tumor.

catamenial migraine. A unique type of migraine suffered by women that occurs at the time of menstruation.

chronic daily headaches. Headaches that occur on a daily basis, usually not migraine headaches.

classic migraine. A migraine headache associated with a warning or premonition, often a vision disturbance.

cluster headaches. A certain type of headache disorder.

common migraine. Migraine headache not associated with a warning or premonition and not associated with any visual disturbance.

diathermy. The use of ice and heat in pain management.

diuretic. Water pill.

emergency headache. A headache that demands emergency attention.

endorphins. The body's natural pain chemicals, produced in the brain.

guided imagery. Similar to hypnosis and breathing techniques; used as a method to adjust the nervous system and produce relaxation.

hypnosis. A unique type of focused attention, often effective in adjusting the body's heart rate, pulse, breathing pattern, and pain levels.

homeopathic medications. Natural chemicals, often available in health food stores and frequently prescribed by holistic or homeopathic physicians; considered natural treatments for various ills.

hypoglycemia. Low blood sugar.

lumbar puncture. Spinal tap; a study used to check the spinal fluid contents to rule out hemorrhage, infection, or cancer.

meningitis. Inflammation and possible infection of the coverings of the brain and spinal cord (as in "spinal meningitis").

migraineur. A patient who suffers from migraine headaches.

monoamine oxidase inhibitors. A class of medicine used to alleviate depression. This class is also often effective in preventing migraine headaches.

MRI. Magnetic resonance imaging scan; a more elaborate image of the brain, which identifies the brain stem, the balance center of the brain, and the small folds of the brain. Scarring and small strokes are often better seen on MRI studies than on CAT scans.

MSG. Monosodium glutamate; one type of food additive that often is a trigger found in multiple foods (please see comments on food restriction and headache disorder).

neural. Pertaining to the nerves and nervous system.

neuro-blockade. Some form of chemical intervention to block the chemical transmitters of the brain and prevent headache.

neurochemical transmission depletion theory. A theory currently held, which is used to explain migraine and its complete spectrum of symptoms.

neurovascular. Pertaining to the nerves and blood vessels in combination.

nonpharmacologic treatments. Treatments for migraine headaches that do not utilize prescription medications.

NSAIDS. Nonsteroidal/anti-inflammatory drugs. Motrin is in this class of drugs, as are many other newer medications.

occipital neuralgia. Inflammation of the nerve at the base of the skull that goes up the back of the head and around the ear. This can lead to sharp, shooting, lacerating pains that can be mistaken for migraine or muscle spasm headaches.

prodrome. The events that precede a migraine headache; often these include nausea, queasiness, vision changes, and throbbing temples.

progressive relaxation. A method of contracting and relaxing a series of muscles in a progressive fashion, producing an overall sense of relaxation and calm.

pseudotumor cerebri. Increased pressure on the brain, often seen in overweight females and often associated with vision problems.

serotonin. A brain chemical that is often implicated in migraine headache disorder.

sinusitis. Inflammation and possible infection of the sinus cavities.

stroke. Loss of blood and oxygen in the brain tissue, which leads to a loss of function related to that area of brain damage (such as weakness, numbness, clumsiness, loss of speech, or paralysis).

subcutaneous. Beneath the skin.

temporal arteritis. Inflammation of the arteries at the sides of the head. If left untreated, can lead to blindness.

tension headaches. The older term for muscle spasm/muscle contraction type headaches. These may be worse when the patient is under stress.

therapeutic massage. A unique type of massage that improves muscle spasm and contraction, as well as muscle inflammation, and is often effective for reducing muscle contraction and mixed headache disorders.

thermography. A temperature study of the brain.

TMJ. Temporomandibular joint dysfunction; these jaw joint problems may be related to headache pains.

transcranial doppler. A non-invasive ultrasound study of the brain's blood vessels.

trigeminal neuralgia. Often referred to as tic douloureaux; this is a brain stem nerve which causes pain in the face and can be confused with migraine or other types of headache pain.

trigger. An item or event that leads to a migraine headache.

tumor. An abnormal growth somewhere in the body, potentially a cancer growth.

tyramine. Chemical substance that acts as a potential chemical transmitter of the brain; may play a role in migraine headaches.

vascular. Pertaining to blood vessels.

visual aura. The flashes of light that precede a migraine headache.

Bibliography

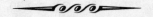

Alvarez, W. C. "The migrainous scotoma as studies in 618 persons." *American Journal of Ophthalmology*, 49:489–504, 1960.

American Academy of Allergy and Immunology. "Candidiasis hypersensitivity syndrome." *Journal of Allergy and Clinical Immunology*, 78:271–273, 1986.

Anthony, M. "Headache and the greater occipital nerve." *Clinical Neurology and Neurosurgery*, 94:297–301, 1992.

Appenzeller, O. "Pathogenesis of migraine (review)." *Medical Clinics of North America*, 75 (3):763–89, May 1991.

Axon, M., et al. "Migraine angitis precipitated by sex headache and leading to watershed infarction." *Cephalgia*, 13:427–30, 1993.

Balch, J. F., et al. *Prescription for Nutritional Healing*. Garden City Park, New York: Avery Publishing Group, 1990.

Barlow, C. F. *Headaches and Migraines in Children*. Oxford: Spastics International Medical Publications, 1984.

Barnard, N. *Power of Your Plate*. Summer-Town, Tennessee: Book Publishing Company, 1990.

Baumel, B., et al. "Diagnosis and treatment of headache in the elderly." *Medical Clinics of North America,* 75:661–675, 1991.

Belgrade, M. J., et al. "Comparison of single dose Meperidine, Butorphanol, and Dihydroergotamine in the treatment of vascular headache." *Neurology,* 39:590–592, 1989.

Blanchard, E. B. "Behavioral therapies in the treatment of headache." *Headache Quarterly: Current Treatment and Research,* 1:53–56, 1993.

Blau, J. N. "How to take a history of head or facial pain." *British Medical Journal,* 285:9–1251, October 30, 1982.

Blau, J. N., et al. "The site of pain origin during migraine attacks." *Cephalgia,* 1:143–7.

Boggs, J. G., et al. "Migraine in liver transplant patients." *Neurology,* 45 (supplement 4):A366, April 1995.

Bradley, Walter G., et al. *Neurology and Clinical Practice.* Boston: Butterworth-Heinmann, 1991.

Buring, J. E., et al. "Migraine and subsequent risk of stroke in the physician's health study." *Neurology,* 52:129–134, 1995.

Cantor, T. G. "Pharmacology and Mechanisms of Some Pain Relieving Drugs," *Headache Quarterly.* February 1988, 61–62.

Cantrell-Simmons, E., et al. "A review of studies on the relationship of chronic analgesic use in chronic headaches." *Headache Quarterly,* 4:28–35, 1993.

Carlsson, J., et al. "Muscle tenderness in tension headache treated with acupuncture or physiotherapy." *Cephalgia,* 10:131–41, 1990.

Castleman, M. *The healing herbs.* Emmaus, PA: Rodale Press, 1991.

Coyle, P. K. "Neurologic complications of Lyme disease and neurologic aspects of rheumatic disease." *Rheumatic Disease Clinics of North America,* 19(4):993–1009, November 1993.

Cronen, M. C., et al. "Cervical steroid epidural nerve block in the palliation of pain secondary to intractable muscle contraction headache." *Headache,* 28:314–315, 1988.

Cummings, Stephen, M.D., and Ullman, Dana, M.P.H. *Everybody's Guide to Homeopathic Medicines.* New York: Jeremy P. Tarcher/Putnam Book, 1991.

Dahlof, M. D., Ph.D., Ekbaum, K., M.D., Ph.D., and Persson, Lennart, M.D., Ph.D. "Clinical Experiences from Sweden on the Use of Subcutaneously Administered Sumatriptan in Migraine and Cluster Headache." *Archives of Neurology*, 51:1256–1261, December 1994.

Dalessio, D. J., et al. *Wolf's headache and other head pain.* Sixth Ed., New York: The University Press, 1993.

Dalessio, D. J. "On the safety of caffeine as an analgesic adjuvant." *Headache Quarterly: Current Treatment and Research*, 5(2):125–127, 1994.

Davidoff, R. A. *Migraine: Manifestations, pathogenesis and management.* Davis Company of Philadelphia, 1995.

DeMatteis, G., et al. "Geomagnetic activity, humidity, temperature and headache: Is there any correlation?" *Headache*, 34:41–43, 1994.

Diamond, S. "Diagnosis and treatment of migraine." *Clinical Journal of Pain*, 5:3–9, 1989.

Diamond S., et al. "Transnasal Butorphanol in the treatment of Migraine Head Pain." *Headache Quarterly*, 3:160–167, 1992.

Drugs for Migraine. *The Medical Letter*, 37 (issue 943):17–20, March 3, 1995.

Ducro, P. N., et al. "Migraine as a sequel to chronic low back pain." *Headache*, 34:279–281, 1994.

Eger, J., et al. "Effective diet treatment on anuresis in children with migraine or hyperkinetic behavior." *Clinical Pediatrics*, (Philadelphia) 5:302–7, May 31, 1992.

Ermenda, P. D., et al. "Extracranial vascular changes as a source of pain in migraine headache." *Annals of Neurology*, 13:32–37, 1983.

Ferrari, M. D., et al. "Treatment of migraine attacks with Sumatriptan." *New England Journal of Medicine*, 325:316–321, 1991.

Ferrari, M. D., et al. "Cerebral blood flow during migraine attacks without aura and effect of Sumatriptan." *Neurology*, 52:135–139, 1995.

Freschi, Joseph R., "Why Migraine Headaches," *Total Health*, 15(6): 36 (2), December 1993.

Friberg, L., et al. "Cerebral oxygen extraction, oxygen consumption, and regional cerebral blood flow during the aura phase of migraine." *Stroke*, 25:974–979. 1994.

Gauthier, J., et al. "The role of home practice in the thermal biofeedback treatment of migraine headache." *Consult Clinical Psychology*, 62 (1):180–4, February 1994.

George, M. S. "Is migraine related to eating disorders?" International Journal of Eating Disorders, 14 (1):75–9, July 1993.

Good, P. A., et al. "The use of tinted glasses in childhood migraine." *Headache*, 31:533–536, 1991.

Goulart, F. S. "The headache alternative: Fifteen natural pain-pain-go-away solutions." *Total Health*, 16, N3: 26 (3), June 1994.

Grazzi, L., et al. "Italian experience of electromyographic biofeedback treatment of episodic common migraine: Preliminary results." *Headache*, 33:439–441, 1993.

Hainline, Brian. "Headache." *Neurologic Clinics*, 12 (3), August 1994 (neurologic complications of pregnancy, 443–459).

Hay, K. M., et al. "1044 women with migraine: The effect of environmental stimuli." *Headache*, March 1994, 166–194.

HEADway, "Now there is MMS: Menstrual Migraine Syndrome." *Newsletter for migraine sufferers*, vol. 3.

Hofert, M. J. "Treatment of migraine: A new era (review)." *American Family Physician*, 49 (3):633-8, 643–4, February 15, 1994.

Igarashi, M., et al. "Pharmacologic treatment of childhood migraine (review)." *Journal of Pediatrics*, 120 (4, Part I):653–7, April 1992.

Inan, L. E., et al. "Complicated retinal migraine." *Headache*, 34:50–52, 1994.

Jensen, R. "Sodium valproate has a prophylactic effect in migraine without aura, a triple blind placebo-controlled crossover study." *Neurology*, 44:647–651, 1994.

Johnson, E. S., et al. "Efficacy of feverfew as prophylactic treatment of migraine." *British Medical Journal*, 291:569–73, 1985.

Jorgensen H. S., et al. "Headache And Stroke: The Copenhagen Stroke Study." *Neurology*, 44:1793–1797, 1994

Kudro, L. "Paradoxical effects of frequent analgesic use." *Advances in Neurology*, 33, 1982, 335–341.

Lake, A. E., et al. "Comprehensive inpatient treatment for intractable migraine: A prospective long-term outcome study." *Headache,* 33 (2):55–62, February 1993.

Lance, F. "Does analgesic abuse cause headaches de novo?" *Headache,* February 1988, 61–62.

Lauritzen, M. "Pathophysiology of the migraine aura. The spreading depression sere (review)." *Brain,* 117 (Part I):199–210, February 1994.

Linet, M. S., et al. "An epidemiologic study of headache in adolescents and young adults." *JAMA,* 261:2211–2216, 1989.

Liu, G. T., et al. "Persistent positive visual phenomena in migraine." *Neurology,* 45:664–668, 1995.

Lundberg, P. O. "Abdominal migraine—Diagnosis and therapy." *Headache,* 15:122–125, 1975.

Mahaja, A. N., et al. "Platelet phospholipase inhibitor from the medicinal herb feverfew (tan-nacetum parthenium), prostaglandins, leukotrienes," *Medicine,* 8:653–60, 1982.

Mansfield, L. "Food allergy and migraine: Double blind and mediator confirmation of an allergic etiology." *Annals of Allergy,* 55:92; 126–129, 1985.

Matthew, N. "Valproate in the treatment of persistent chronic daily headache." *Headache,* 30:301,1990.

Mauskop, A. "Chronic daily headache—One disease or two? Diagnostic role of serum ionized magnesium." *Cephalgia,* 14 (1):24–8, February 1994.

Mauskop, Alexander, et al. "Intravenous (IV) magnesium sulfate (MgSO4) relieves acute migraine (M) in patients (P) with low serum ionized magnesium levels (IMG2+)." *Neurology,* 45 (supplement 4), p. A379, April 1995.

McGrady, A., et al. "Effective biofeedback—assisted relaxation on migraine headache and changes of cerebral blood flow velocity in the middle cerebral artery." *Headache,* 34 (7):424–8, July-August 1994.

Mortimer, M. J., et al. "The prevalence of headache and migraine in atopic children: An epidemiologic study in general practice." *Headache,* 33 (8):427–31, September 1993.

Moskowitz, M. A. "Brain mechanisms in vascular headache." *Neurologic Clinics*, 8:801–815, 1990.

Nappi, Giuseppe. "Oral Sumatriptan compared with placebo in the acute treatment of migraine." *Journal of Neurology*, 241:138–144, 1994.

Neurologic Clinics: Headache, 1 (2) B. Saunders Co., Russel C. Packard, M.D., Guest Editor, May 1983.

Newman, L. C., Lipton, R. B. and Soloman, S. "Hemicrania Continua: Ten New Cases in Review of the Literature." *Neurology*, 44: 2111–2114, 1994.

Nicolodi, M., et al. "Visceral pain threshold is deeply lowered far from the head in migraine." *Headache*, 34:12-19, 1994.

Niedermeyer, E. "Migraine-Triggered Epilepsy." *Clinical Electro-encephalography*, 24: 37–43, 1993.

Oldman, B. "Chronic pain and the search for alternative treatments." *Medical Association Journal*, 145 (5):508–513, 1991.

Olesen, J. "Understanding the biologic basis of migraine." *New England Journal of Medicine*, 331 (25) ; 1713–1714.

Osipova, V. "Psycho-autonomic approaches to migraine." *Functional Neurology*, 7 (4):263–73, July-August 1992.

Osterhaus, J. T., et al. "Health care resource and lost labor costs of migraine headache in the United States." *Pharmaco-economics*, 2:67–76, 1992.

Ottman, R. and Lipton, R. B. "Comorbidity of Migraine and Epilepsy." *Neurology*, 44: 2105–2110, 1994.

Packard, R. C. "Emotional aspects of headache." *Neurologic Clinics: Symposium on Headache*, 1:445–456, 1983.

Panayiotopoulos, C. P. "Elementary visual hallucinations in migraine and epilepsy." *Journal of Neurology, Neurosurgery and Psychiatry*, 57:1371–1374, 1994.

Pareja, J. A., et al. "Sunct syndrome in the female." *Headache*, 34:217–220, 1994.

Passchier, J. "A critical note on psycho-physiological stress research into migraine patients (review article)." *Cephalgia*, 3:194–8, 1984.

Perlmutter, D. *Life Guide—Your guide to a longer and healthier life."* Vol. 1, 2nd ed. Naples, Florida: Life Guide Press, 1994.

Perneger, T. V., et al. "Risk of kidney failure associated with the use of acetaminophen, aspirin, and nonsteroidal/anti-inflammatory drugs." *New England Journal of Medicine,* 331:167–9, 1994.

Pradaliera, et al. "Treatment review: Nonsteroidal/anti-inflammatory drugs in treatment and long-term prevention of migraine attacks." *Headache,* 28:550–557, 1988.

Raskin, N. H. "Repetitive intravenous Dihydroergotamine for the treatment of intractable migraine." *Neurology,* 34:245, 1984.

Raskin, N. H. "Acute and prophylactic treatment of migraine: Practical approaches and pharmacological rationale (review)." *Neurology,* 43 (6 supplement 3):S39–42, June 1993.

Raskin, N. H. "Headache (review)." *Western Journal of Medicine,* 161 (3):299–302, September 1994.

Reik, L. "Lyme disease—Current therapy." In R. Johnson, M.D. (ed.), *Neurologic Disease,* 3rd ed. textbook. Philadelphia: B. C. Decker, 1990.

Robbins, L. D. "Cryotherapy for headache." *Headache,* 29:598–600, 1989.

Robbins, L. "Precipitating factors in migraine: A retrospective review of 494 patients." *ACHE,* pp. 214–216, April 1994.

Sacks, Oliver. *Migraine: Evolution of a Common Disorder.* Berkeley: University of California Press, 1970.

Schesse, J. "Acupuncture vs. Metoprolol in migraine prophylaxis: A randomized trial of trigger point inactivation." *Journal of Internal Medicine,* 235:451-456, 1994.

Schulman, E. A., et al. "Symptomatic and prophylactic treatment of migraine and tension type headache (review)." *Neurology,* 42 (3 supplement 2):16–21, March 1992.

Shadick, N. A., et al. "The long-term clinical outcomes of Lyme disease." *Annals of Internal Medicine,* 121:560–567, 1994.

Smeets, M. C. "Intracellular and plasma magnesium in familial hemiplegic migraine and migraine with and without aura." *Cephalgia,* 14 (1):29–32, February 1994.

Soloman, S., et al. "Breaking the cycle of pain." *Medical World News,* December 1993.

Stewart, W. F., et al. "Prevalence of migraine headache." *JAMA,* 267 (1): 64–69, January 1, 1992.

Stewart, W. F., Ph.D, M.P.H. "Impact of Migraine." *Neurology,* 44 (Supplement 4): S 5, 1994.

Stewart, W. F., Ph.D., M.P.H., "Migraine Prevalence: A Review of Population-Based Studies," *Neurology,* 44 (supplement 4): S 17–23, 1994.

Subcutaneous Sumatriptan International Study Group, "Treatment of migraine attacks with Sumatriptan." *New England Journal of Medicine,* 325:316-327, 1991.

Silberstein, S. D. "Headaches in women: Treatment of the pregnant and lactating migraineur." *Headache,* 33:533–540, 1993.

Solomon, G. D. "Pharmacology and use of headache medications." *Cleveland Clinic Journal of Medicine,* 57:627–635, 1990.

Silvestrini, M., et al. "Migraine in patients with stroke and anti-phospholipid antibodies." *Headache,* 33:421–426, 1993.

Sjaastad, O. O., et al. "Cervicogenic headache; the differentiation from common migraine. An overview." *Functional Neurology,* 6 (2): 93–99, 1991.

Somerville, B. W. "A study of migraine in pregnancy." *Neurology,* 22:824–828, 1972.

Strom, B. L. "Adverse reactions to over-the-counter analgesics taken for therapeutic purposes." *JAMA,* 272 (23): 1866–1867, December 21, 1994.

Touchon, J., et al. "A comparison of SC Sumatriptan and intranasal Dihydroergotamine (DHE) in the treatment of migraine." *Neurology,* 45 (supplement 4): A378, April 1995.

Trotsky, M. B. "Neurogenic vascular headaches, food, and chemical triggers." *Ears, Nose and Throat Journal,* 73 (4): 228–30, 235–6, April 1994.

Value of heat and ice therapy (educational bulletin). Gulf Coast Spine Institute, May 1995.

Vaughan, T. R. "The role of food in the pathogenesis of migraine headache." *Clinical Review of Allergy,* 12 (2):167–80, Summer 1994.

Vijayan, N. "Head band for migraine headache relief." *Headache,* 33:40–42, 1993.

Vincent, C. A. "The treatment of tension headache by acupuncture: A controlled single case designed with time series analysis." *Journal of Psychosomatic Research*, 34 (5): 553–561, 1990.

Weiss, E., and English, O. S. *Psychosomatic Medicine*, 2nd Ed., Saunders, 1949.

Whitcomb, D. C., et al. "Association of acetaminophen hepatotoxicity with fasting and ethanol abuse." *JAMA*, 272:1845–1850, 1994.

Wilkinson, M. "Migraine treatment: The British perspective (Magnesium in migraine. Results in a multicenter pilot study), *Fortschr Medizin*, 112 (24):328–30, August 30, 1994.

Wilson, J., et al. "Spreading cerebral oligemia in classical and normal cerebral blood flow in common migraine." *Headache*, 22:242–249.

Woods, R. P., et al. "Bilateral spreading cerebral hypoperfusion during spontaneous migraine headache." *New England Journal of Medicine*, 31 (25):1689–1692, November 22, 1994.

Yuanm. "Clinical application of point-through-point acupuncture." *Journal of Traditional Chinese Medicine*, 12.

Ziegler, D. K. "Dihydroergotamine nasal spray for the acute treatment of migraine." *Neurology*, 44:447-453, 1994.

Ziegler, D. K. "Dihydroergotamine nasal spray." *Neurology*, 45.

Index

Health Care in
Orient Paperbacks

Complete Family Medicine Book	Drs. Dandiya & Bapna	
Homoeopathic Remedies for Infants and Children	Dr. Sudha Bannerjee	Rs. 125
Homoeopathic Remedies for Middle and Old Age	Dr. Keith Souter	Rs. 110
Healing Power of Garlic	Paul Bergner	Rs. 110
Asthma Self-Help Book *(illus.)*	Dr. Paul J. Hannaway	Rs. 110
Exercising for a Healthy Heart *(illus.)*	Dr. Paul Vodak	Rs. 70
Hot Water Therapy *(illus.)*	Dr. Patrik & D. Harp	Rs. 75
Herbal Remedies & Home Comforts	Jill Nice	Rs. 80
Fitness Walking *(illus.)*	Snowdon & Humphreys	Rs. 90
Yogic Pranayama: Breathing for Long Life & Good Health *(illus.)*	Dr. K.S. Joshi	Rs. 90
Cure Aches & Pains Through Osteopathy	Dr. K.M. Modi	Rs. 90
Conquering Backpain *(illus.)*	Donald Norfolk	Rs. 90
Vitamins That Heal	H.K. Bakhru	Rs. 55
Foods That Heal	H.K. Bakhru	Rs. 55
Yogic Cure for Common Diseases	Dr. Phulgenda Sinha	Rs. 45
Magnetic Cure for Common Diseases *(illus.)*	Dr. H.L. Bansal	Rs. 45
Ayurvedic Cure for Common Diseases *(illus.)*	Dr. N.A. Murthy & D.P. Pandey	Rs. 50
High Blood Cholesterol: Causes, Prevention & Treatment *(illus.)*	Dr. Krishan Gupta	Rs. 50
Diabetes: Causes, Prevention & Treatment *(illus.)*	Ada P. Kahn	Rs. 45

Available at all bookshops or by VPP

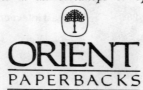

ORIENT
PAPERBACKS

Madarsa Rd, Kashmere Gate
Delhi - 110 006. India